Risking Intimacy and Creative Transformation in Psychoanalysis

In this compelling book, Lauren Levine explores the transformative power of stories and storytelling in psychoanalysis to heal psychic wounds and create shared symbolic meaning and coherence out of ungrieved loss and trauma.

Through evocative clinical stories, Levine considers the impact of trauma and creativity on the challenge of creating one's own story, resonant with personal authenticity and a shared sense of culture and history. Levine sees creativity as an essential aspect of aliveness, and as transformative, emergent in the clinical process. She utilizes film, dance, poetry, literature, and dreams as creative frames to explore diverse aspects of psychoanalytic process. As a psychoanalyst and writer, Levine is interested in the stories we tell, individually and collectively, as well as what gets disavowed and dissociated by experiences of relational, intergenerational, and sociopolitical trauma. She is concerned too with whose stories get told and whose get erased, silenced, and marginalized. This crucial question, what gets left out of the narrative, and the potential for an intimate psychoanalytic process to help patients reclaim what has been lost, is at the heart of this volume.

Attentive to the work of helping patients reclaim their memory and creative agency, this book will prove invaluable for psychoanalysts and psychotherapists in practice and in training.

Lauren Levine is joint Editor-in-Chief of *Psychoanalytic Dialogues*. She teaches and presents both nationally and internationally, and has published articles about sociocultural, racial and relational trauma, resilience, and creativity. Dr. Levine is faculty at the NYU Postdoctoral Program in Psychoanalysis, and the Stephen Mitchell Relational Study Center, where she is codirector of the One Year Program in Relational Studies. She is visiting faculty at the Institute for Relational and Group Psychotherapy in Athens, Greece, and the Tampa Bay Psychoanalytic Society, and supervisor at the Institute for Relational Psychoanalysis of Philadelphia. Dr. Levine is a psychoanalyst in private practice in New York City.

Relational Perspectives Book Series

Adrienne Harris & Eyal Rozmarin
Series Editors

Stephen Mitchell
Founding Editor

Lewis Aron
Editor Emeritus

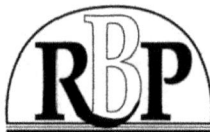

The Relational Perspectives Book Series (RPBS) publishes books that grow out of or contribute to the relational tradition in contemporary psychoanalysis. The term *relational psychoanalysis* was first used by Greenberg and Mitchell[1] to bridge the traditions of interpersonal relations, as developed within interpersonal psychoanalysis and object relations, as developed within contemporary British theory. But, under the seminal work of the late Stephen A. Mitchell, the term *relational psychoanalysis* grew and began to accrue to itself many other influences and developments. Various tributaries—interpersonal psychoanalysis, object relations theory, self psychology, empirical infancy research, feminism, queer theory, sociocultural studies and elements of contemporary Freudian and Kleinian thought—flow into this tradition, which understands relational configurations between self and others, both real and fantasied, as the primary subject of psychoanalytic investigation.

We refer to the relational tradition, rather than to a relational school, to highlight that we are identifying a trend, a tendency within contemporary psychoanalysis, not a more formally organized or coherent school or system of beliefs. Our use of the term *relational* signifies a dimension of theory and practice that has become salient across the wide spectrum of contemporary psychoanalysis. Now under the editorial supervision of Adrienne Harris and Eyal Rozmarin, the Relational Perspectives Book Series originated in 1990 under the editorial eye of the late Stephen A. Mitchell. Mitchell was the most prolific and influential of the originators of the relational tradition. Committed to dialogue among psychoanalysts, he abhorred the authoritarianism that dictated adherence to a rigid set of beliefs or technical restrictions. He championed open discussion, comparative and integrative approaches, and promoted new voices across the generations. Mitchell was later joined by the late Lewis Aron, also a visionary and influential writer, teacher and leading thinker in relational psychoanalysis.

Included in the Relational Perspectives Book Series are authors and works that come from within the relational tradition, those that extend and develop that tradition, and works that critique relational approaches or compare and contrast them with alternative points of view. The series includes our most distinguished senior psychoanalysts, along with younger contributors who bring fresh vision. Our aim is to enable a deepening of relational thinking while reaching across disciplinary and social boundaries in order to foster an inclusive and international literature.

A full list of titles in this series is available at https://www.routledge.com/Relational-Perspectives-Book-Series/book-series/LEARPBS.

Note

1 Greenberg, J. & Mitchell, S. (1983). *Object relations in psychoanalytic theory*. Cambridge, MA: Harvard University Press.

'In this exquisite new book, Lauren Levine captures the finely nuanced tapestry that emerges when an analytic dyad takes shape; the interweaving of two different narratives of self that come together, engage with each other, distance each other and ultimately form the subject matter of the analysis that unfolds. With brilliant clarity, and detailed and forthrightly honest clinical examples, Levine demonstrates how the collision of the patient's and the analyst's preferred life stories demands the analyst's, at times painful emotional honesty, in re-opening dissociated pockets of enlivening engagement and creativity.'

Jody Messler Davies, *NYU Postdoctoral Program,*
Stephen Mitchell Center for Relational Studies

'In this powerful and creative volume, *Risking Intimacy and Creative Transformation in Psychoanalysis*, Lauren Levine explores the healing power of stories as they touch our vulnerabilities, our strengths and resilience, intrapsychic and sociocultural traumas. Levine beautifully explores the transformative value of sharing our stories with a listening, witnessing other, bearing witness to our wounds, our shame, and our collective sins.'

Galit Atlas, *author of* Emotional Inheritance;
NYU Postdoctoral Program in Psychoanalysis

'*Risking Intimacy and Creative Transformation in Psychoanalysis* is a wonder, a collection of essays whose honesty, integrity and authenticity challenge us and teach us, making us more vulnerable and hence more alive than we were before reading. It provides a relational blueprint to the intricacies of our deepest fears and fantasies about the psychoanalytic process as well as an openness to the insidious impact of racism and sociopolitical trauma. It is extremely rare that such a broad range of the human experience is taken on by any author; it is a rarity indeed for it to be done with such brilliance, thoughtfulness and creative care. This is a most welcome book, which should be read and re-read for the often painful aliveness it brings to the therapeutic encounter.'

Steve Tuber, *author of* Attachment, Play and Authenticity:
Winnicott in Clinical Context

'In this moving and incisive work, Lauren Levine reminds us that storytelling has both dangerous and curative dimensions. We often use stories to evade our own traumas and hide from self-awareness the gaps in our personal narratives. This has also been true of the field, in terms of the stories psychoanalysts feel comfortable engaging in our various models of the psyche. With an emphasis on the *sharing* of stories as the key to transformative mental healing, *Risking Intimacy and Creative Transformation* offers a powerful introduction to the insights of a relational psychoanalysis that can address the racial and cultural traumas of the 21st century.'

Michelle Stephens, *founding executive director, Institute for the Study of Global Racial Justice, professor of English and Latino and Caribbean Studies, Rutgers University*

'Lauren Levine explores the creative potential of what might be called story living. She captures how shared stories build relational and political transformations. But only, as Levine carefully details, when patient and analyst together confront personal inhibitions and cultural prohibitions that render stories normotic and deadening. Levine theorizes and clinically animates the ways in which we not only "tell ourselves stories in order to live," as per Didion, but also how we tell stories to change the order of living.'

Ken Corbett, *NYU Postdoctoral Program in Psychoanalysis and Psychotherapy*

'Lauren Levine's highly creative work, *Risking Intimacy and Creative Transformation in Psychoanalysis*, marks the evolution of relational theory as a space of increasingly wonderful complexity. Her clinical and theoretical approach stresses the role of imagination and novel forms of clinical interaction. In this work, weaving film, poetry and dance into compelling psychoanalytic stories, we see both clinical and theoretical movement and expansion.'

Adrienne Harris, *NYU Postdoctoral Program in Psychoanalysis and New School for Social Research*

Risking Intimacy and Creative Transformation in Psychoanalysis

Lauren Levine

Routledge
Taylor & Francis Group

LONDON AND NEW YORK

Designed cover image: Great Island Sunset – Sunspots, acrylic on panel, 16" x 20", copyright Rowena Perkins, 2022
Rowenaperkinsstudio.com

First published 2023
by Routledge
4 Park Square, Milton Park, Abingdon, Oxon OX14 4RN

and by Routledge
605 Third Avenue, New York, NY 10158

Routledge is an imprint of the Taylor & Francis Group, an informa business

© 2023 Lauren Levine

British Library Cataloguing-in-Publication Data
A catalogue record for this book is available from the British Library

ISBN: 978-1-032-43470-4 (hbk)
ISBN: 978-1-032-43474-2 (pbk)
ISBN: 978-1-003-36747-5 (ebk)

DOI: 10.4324/9781003367475

Typeset in Times New Roman
by MPS Limited, Dehradun

Contents

Acknowledgments

First and foremost, I want to thank Adrienne Harris, my writing mentor, supervisor, treasured colleague, and friend of many years. I could not have written this book without you and your creativity, inspiration, and support, as well as the care and imagination of our writing group with Bob Bartlett, Kirsten Lentz, and Rachel Kozlowski, and previously with Julia Beltsiou. Huge thanks to you all.

To my dear friends and joint editors-in-chief of *Psychoanalytic Dialogues*, Stephen Hartman, Jack Foehl and Amy Schwartz Cooney, I am enormously grateful to U3 for your support of my writing, and for the opportunity to co-lead the journal, building on and expanding the radical inquiry and generative dialogues of relational psychoanalysis.

A big thank you to the prior editors of *Psychoanalytic Dialogues*, Tony Bass, Hazel Ipp, and Stephen Seligman, for your meaningful support and friendship. And a special thank you to Tony, my first supervisor and mentor at NYU Postdoc, who edited and supported my writing and professional development over many years.

To Lew Aron and Philip Bromberg, vital and inspiring mentors whom I miss deeply, thank you for your wisdom, creativity, and vision, and for your faith in me and encouragement of my writing.

To Anita Herron, my suite-mate and codirector of the One Year Program in Relational Studies at the Stephen Mitchell Center, thank you for your creative collaboration in envisioning a broader, more inclusive curriculum attentive to the sociocultural and intersectional context of relational psychoanalysis.

This book would not have been possible without the support of so many dear friends and colleagues including: Lycia Guerra Alexander, Pam Allyn, Rachel Altstein, Shari Appollon, Maria Paz Ardito, Kelly Arteaga, Galit Atlas, Laura Benkov, Andrea Rihm Bianchi, Donna Brindle, Velleda Ceccoli, Stavros Charambides, Steven Cooper, Ken Corbett, Jody Davies, Deborah Dowd, Janine de Peyer, Gordon Fearey, my Aunt Harriet Feiner, Heather Ferguson, Mark Gerald, Stefanie Solow Glennon, Susan Greenfield, Rachel Kabasakalian McKay, Matina Kaidantzi, Alan Kintzer, Lorraine Kushner, Maria Lechich, Hilary Levine, Patricia Martin, Belkis Martinez, Charla Melamed, Sarah Mendelsohn, Spyros Orfanos, Ieasha Ramsay, Judy Roth, Peter Rudnytsky, Marie Saba, Sarah Schoen, Eben Shapiro, Sandy Silverman, Mark Singer, David Spound, Michelle Stephens, Melanie Suchet, Steve Tuber, and Kirkland Vaughans.

A special thank you to Darlene Ehrenberg. For so many reasons.

I am grateful to my colleagues, supervisees, and students at NYU Postdoc and the Stephen Mitchell Center, and appreciative of the International Association for Relational Psychotherapy and Psychoanalysis, Division 39 of the APA, the Institute for Relational and Group Psychotherapy in Athens, Greece, the Tampa Bay Psychoanalytic Society, and the Boston Psychoanalytic Society and Institute who have invited me to teach and play and present and have engaged enthusiastically with my work over many years.

Huge thanks to Kate Hawes and Georgina Clutterbuck, my publishers at Taylor and Francis, for believing in me and my writing and ushering me through the publishing process with such warmth, encouragement, and generosity. Thanks also to the design team led by Jo Griffin and the wider production team led by Sian Cahill.

Thank you to my friend, Rowena Perkins, artist extraordinaire, for the photograph of your gorgeous painting, *Great Island Sunset—Sunspots,* that graces my book cover.

To Jeannie Blaustein, my dearest friend of 40 years, thank you for being you, and being right there, always, through the darkness and the light. Love you.

Being a psychoanalyst is a great privilege, and I am most appreciative of my patients, who have trusted me and allowed me to join them on our unique and mutually transformative journeys. I have learned so much from each of you. And to my patients who have given me permission to share our stories in these chapters, I am especially grateful.

Finally, my deepest love and gratitude to Linda and Larry, Hilary and Audrey, and of course, Jesse, Daniel, and Jim.

Credits List

Earlier versions of five of these chapters were previously published in *Psychoanalytic Dialogues*, and are gratefully reprinted here by permission of the publisher:

- Lauren Levine (2009) Transformative Aspects of Our Own Analyses and Their Resonance in Our Work with Our Patients, Psychoanalytic Dialogues, 19:4, 454–462, DOI: 10.1080/10481880903088641. https://www.tandfonline.com/
- Lauren Levine (2012) Into Thin Air: The Co-Construction of Shame, Recognition, and Creativity in an Analytic Process, Psychoanalytic Dialogues, 22:4, 456–471, DOI: 10.1080/10481885.2012.701140. https://www.tandfonline.com/
- Lauren Levine (2016) A Mutual Survival of Destructiveness and Its Creative Potential for Agency and Desire, Psychoanalytic Dialogues, 26:1, 36–49, DOI: 10.1080/10481885.2016.1123511. https://www.tandfonline.com/
- Lauren Levine (2016) Mutual Vulnerability: Intimacy, Psychic Collisions, and the Shards of Trauma, Psychoanalytic Dialogues, 26:5, 571–579, DOI: 10.1080/10481885.2016.1214471. https://www.tandfonline.com/
- Lauren Levine (2022) Interrogating Race, Shame and Mutual Vulnerability: Overlapping and Interlapping Waves of Relation, Psychoanalytic Dialogues, 32:2, 99–113, DOI: 10.1080/10481885.2022.2033546. https://www.tandfonline.com/

Introduction

In this book, I explore the transformative power of stories and storytelling, the power of stories to heal, to create shared symbolic meaning and coherence out of ungrieved loss and trauma. I consider the impact of trauma and creativity on the challenge of creating one's own coherent story, one resonant with both personal authenticity and a shared sense of culture and history. As a psychoanalyst and writer, I am interested in the stories we tell, individually and collectively, as well as what gets *left out* of the narrative, the gaps and holes; what gets disavowed, dissociated, and disrupted by experiences of relational, intergenerational, and sociopolitical trauma.

In her book, *Create Dangerously: The Immigrant Artist at Work*, the Haitian novelist and essayist, Edwidge Danticat (2011) asks "What happens when we cannot tell our stories, when our memories have abandoned us" (p. 65)? This crucial question is at the heart of my book. When one cannot tell one's own stories, when one's memories have been forsaken, working to reclaim one's memory and creative agency becomes a central task of psychoanalysis, making sense of one's personal and sociocultural history, and becoming the storyteller of one's own life. Danticat writes that creating dangerously means, "creating as a revolt against silence, creating when both the creation and the reception, the writing and the reading, are dangerous undertakings" (p. 11).

This notion of *creating dangerously* strikes me as a powerful metaphor for psychoanalysis, as well as art and writing, involving creativity and generativity, the courage to take risks, to challenge orthodoxy and normativity. Creating as a revolt against silence holds

DOI: 10.4324/9781003367475-1

dense meaning in terms of the danger of telling one's story, of making the private, public. Trusting an Other to listen, to respond with compassion and understanding when one has been traumatized, when the menacing message of the perpetrator was to silence or threaten, entails profound peril. We know from Ferenczi, who believed his patients' stories of rape and sexual abuse were real, not fantasies, and understood the doubled, devastating trauma and gaslighting that occurs when one's reality is questioned, or when one is blamed for the abuse. Having the courage to allow one's authentic voices to emerge and not being met or recognized can lead to enormous shame and despair. The challenge, for those who have experienced overwhelming trauma, becomes how to open access to unbearable affects in a relationship that feels safe enough, to breathe life and give form and meaning to the frozen, dissociated, not-me remnants, so that one can begin to feel less ashamed and humiliated of those split-off, unacceptable parts of oneself (e.g., Bromberg, Davies, Dowd, Harris, Levine, Mendelsohn).

Perhaps creating dangerously has particular resonance for Relational psychoanalysis, which was built on radical inquiry, querying Classical assumptions about analytic knowing, authority, and neutrality. Psychoanalysis entails dangerous undertakings for the analyst as well as the patient, as there is vulnerability in being a listener, a witness, a traveling companion, and a co-writer of the story. Throughout the book, I investigate ways in which as analysts, our own relational stories, what Adrienne Harris calls, "our wounds that must serve as tools," (Harris, 2009) represent both our greatest liability and most powerful resource, at times facilitating, and at times impeding our capacity to engage deeply in the analytic process. This has been a central theme for me in my work and in my writing, the challenges and creative potential of this *mutual vulnerability*, the ways in which, as analysts, we are penetrated by shards of our patients' trauma, which flow through and through us, haunting and dysregulating, colliding and interpenetrating with our own vulnerabilities and losses (Aron, Bass, 2015; Harris, 2009; Levine, 2009, 2016b).

I was thrilled to discover the writing of French psychoanalyst and philosopher Anne Dufourmantelle through Chilean colleagues (Maria Paz Ardito and Andrea Rihm, personal communication) who are part of a feminist, psychoanalytic collective. Dufourmantelle (2019) writes about the radical act of intimacy, which entails something akin to Ghent's (1990) notion of surrender—the risk of opening oneself to something hidden in both oneself and in the Other, as well as a radical trust in the unknown of what will evolve. It seems to me that this is the essence of psychoanalysis as creating dangerously.

Shame

Sharing one's stories of injury and violation is a radical undertaking. Far from merely telling a story from the past, it's as if one is back in time. Time falls away, and the accompanying affective experiences of terror and shame get reawakened and rush in, re-experienced in the here and now retelling of trauma. This shame-infused experience presents some of our greatest clinical challenges as analysts, described powerfully by Philip Bromberg (2006):

> The most powerful affect a person is unable to modulate is the experience of shame. The patient is feeling overwhelmed, not simply by reliving such traumatic affects from the past, as anger, fear, grief, sadness and futility, but by a dissociated here-and-now shame experience that gets triggered by the analyst's unawareness and seeming indifference to the fact that his therapeutic "success" in bringing about the reliving of unprocessed traumatic affect leaves his patient needing relief but being unable to communicate the need. As in the original trauma, the person from whom a soothing response is needed is the person least likely to offer it on his own, because he is also the person whose behavior is causing the pain. To the degree that the patient's dissociated shame caused by this unaddressed and unprocessed aspect of their ongoing interaction remains unrecognized by the analyst, the threat of re-traumatization looms larger and larger for the patient. (pp. 8–9)

For the analyst, there is vulnerability in being a witness to stories of trauma as shame can travel insidiously across relational realms, passed back and forth, alternately projected and introjected, from patient to analyst and back again, deadening spontaneity, imagination, and creativity (Levine, 2009). With the Relational turn, there has been a theoretical shift in our understanding of shame as inherently intersubjective as well as intrapsychic, which Mitchell referred to as the interpersonalization of shame. As I will illustrate in several chapters, shame can also shut down access to one's creative voice and generative potential and create obstacles to vitality and intimacy in relationships.

However, when shame can be held, reflected upon, and metabolized, it can create an unbinding, an unsettled space, a disruption out of which something new can emerge, making change and creativity possible. Shame can serve as a potential window into new, deeper, and necessary conversations, particularly vis-a-vis race and racism. When shame can be reckoned with, rather than dissociated, it can lead to ethical action, as Lynne Layton (2019) suggests, and to reparation, when inevitable shameful collisions occur. Moving closer into shame, especially what Layton calls, *deserved shame,* entails a willingness to step into vulnerability, a letting go of one's ego, empathizing with, and embracing the experience of the other. Grand (2018) suggests, collective racial shame can feel persecutory, collapsing into violence, denial, or vengeance. OR it "can be a call to conscience, an awakening to social pathologies ... anticipating movement: from moralism to ethics, from solipsism to I-Thou conversation, from denial to collective responsibility" (p. 86).

Mutual Vulnerability

While our work can be deeply satisfying and transformative for the analyst as well as the patient, absorbing our patients' trauma, day in and day out, while we reckon with the challenges in our own lives can take a toll on us as analysts. I think it necessitates an essential porousness, an openness to being deeply penetrated that is an additional burden or hazard of working relationally. Although we have learned so much about mutual vulnerability from Aron, Bass, the Barrangers, Bleger, Ehrenberg, Ferenczi, Searles, and others, less has been written about the importance and complexity of analytic self-care (Corbett, 2012; Harris, 2010). I think we need to be thinking more, and theorizing more, about how we take care of ourselves, as analysts, when we are working in such deep, mutual, and potentially destabilizing ways.

While psychoanalysis has traditionally been conceptualized as a reworking of the past, I will explore ways in which therapeutic change evolves in different registers, layers, and temporalities; a reimagining of the past, as well as envisioning memories from the future (Aron and Atlas, 2015; Bion, 1991; Cooper, 2016a). Our stories connect us to, and help us separate from our ancestors, to our pasts and potential futures. I will illustrate ways in which the edge of growth is inherently vulnerable, nonlinear, and destabilizing. As Seligman (2016) suggests, trauma complicates the process of becoming "a self in time ... a sense of personal security, vital intersubjectivity and temporality ... a sense of moving forward into a lively future" (p. 110–111). Aron and Atlas (2015) propose that it's not just the *working through* of enactments that's potentially generative and transformative, but the flow of enactive engagement in and of itself, as enactments are as "a central means by which patient and analyst enter into each other's inner worlds and discover themselves as participants within each other's psyches" (p. 316). Enactments serve as a rehearsal, a practicing for the future, as well as a working through of the past.

Psychoanalysis has evolved significantly from Freud's archeological notions of stories waiting to be discovered and unearthed, by making the unconscious, conscious, to a model of the story as emergent, evolving, nonlinear, and cocreated (Ferro, Harris, Stern). I am moved by and resonate with Ogden's (2009) description of *rediscovering* psychoanalysis:

> I view it as my role to create psychoanalysis freshly with each patient in each session ... A critically important aspect of this rediscovery of psychoanalysis is the creation of ways of talking with each patient that are unique to that patient in that moment ... I am referring not simply to the unself-conscious use of different tones of voice, rhythms of speech, choice of words, ... but also to particular ways of being with, and communicating with, another person that could exist between no two other people on this planet. (p. 2)

Harris (2009) elaborates on the importance of time and nonlinearity, and the importance of loss and destructiveness in growth and change. She writes:

> Return and repetition are always elements of change; change is, above all, nonlinear, that, in change, time moves in manifold

directions and our experiences, collective, dyadic, or solitary, are always multiply configured ... There is, in efforts to change, an impulse for freedom, always lived with a mixture of exhilaration and destructiveness. There is melancholy and a sense of loss and sadness that weaves through change.

(Harris, 2009, p. 4)

There has been a shift in psychoanalytic understandings of the mind and the nature of unconscious mental processes away from the idea of vertical layers of conscious/ preconscious/unconscious layers per se, "toward a view of the self as decentered, and the mind as a configuration of shifting, nonlinear, discontinuous states of consciousness in an ongoing dialectic with the healthy illusion of unitary selfhood" (Bromberg, 1998, p. 511). Similarly, there's been a shift away from the analyst as the one who knows, the analyst as interpreter of the patient's intrapsychic life to a shift, as Ogden (2019) suggests, from an epistemological model of knowing and understanding to a more ontological model focused on being and becoming:

From the perspective of ontological psychoanalysis, it is not the knowledge arrived at by patient and analyst that is the central point; rather, it is the patient's experience of "arriv[ing] at understanding creatively and with immense joy," an experience in which the patient is engaged not predominantly in searching for self-understanding, but in experiencing the process of becoming more fully himself. (p. 665)

What Gets Left Out of the Stories We Tell

I want to come back to the question I posed earlier, about the importance of the gaps and holes, what gets left out of the stories we tell, and deconstruct Danticat's question: "What happens when we cannot tell our stories, when our memories have abandoned us?" I want to interrogate this question from both an individual and transgenerational perspective about the complexity of trauma, memory, and dissociation, and a larger sociopolitical viewpoint in terms of whose stories get told, centered, embraced as truth, and whose get erased, whitewashed, disappeared from how history is passed down, written and taught.

Abraham (1988) suggests that what haunts us are not *the dead*, but the gaps left within us by the secrets of others. Building on Faimberg's notion of a telescoping of generations, Salberg (2017) suggests that it may take three generations to contain disturbing feelings and events. Unspoken traumatic stories and dissociated affect get passed from one generation to the next, as "parents extrude the traumatic contents of their minds into their children" (p. 78). The novelist Maya Angelou writes: "There is no greater agony than bearing an untold story inside you." The pain leaks out in enigmatic ways. This theme, that the secrets, ghosts, and buried, unprocessed traumas of our ancestors reside in us, and become the legacy carried forward into future generations reverberates throughout Galit Atlas' (2022) book, *Emotional Inheritance*. Atlas writes:

> How do we inherit, hold, and process things that we don't remember or didn't experience ourselves? What is the weight of that which is present but not fully known? Can we really keep secrets from one another, and what do we pass on to the next generation? (p. 12)

The courage to engage deeply in analysis entails a willingness to be unsettled and destabilized by our most wounded patients, reckoning with our own vulnerabilities, nightmares and capacity for destructiveness. It entails casting ourselves into the chaos of our patients' inner worlds by looking into our own wounded hearts; struggling to locate ourselves and our own vulnerabilities in order for our patients to feel deeply seen and recognized. Areas of deep mutual vulnerability can lead to overwhelm or dissociation in the analyst, and can get in the way, at least temporarily, of going deeper into the patient's wounds and unresolved traumas. But openness to our own ghosts, to swimming in uncharted, often frightening territory can potentially unfreeze time and create a renewed sense of vitalization (Schwartz Cooney, 2021), flow, and mutual generativity in analysis (Dowd, 2018; Mendelsohn, 2018).

Collective Trauma and Decentering Whiteness

Historically, just as psychoanalysis began with a focus on the individual and the intrapsychic, the focus of most writing on the intergenerational transmission of trauma was on the impact of a parent's trauma on her child's mind (Abraham and Torok, 1984; Faimberg, 2005; Laub, 2017). There has been much writing on the intergenerational impact of the Holocaust. As Powell (2018) suggests,

> Psychoanalysts have extensively explored the dynamics leading to the Holocaust, mass violence, genocide, and the seeds for within-nation conflicts that result in murderous violence, along with its psychological sequelae in a European context. Less explored is the psychic impact of American slavery on the minds of the nation's inhabitants. (p. 1022)

I am concerned with the racialized and sociocultural trauma that has been dissociated, how whiteness has been the default, and the stories and histories of Black, Indigenous, and other people of color have been marginalized, erased, and disavowed, in this country and within psychoanalysis and in our mostly white analytic institutes (e.g., Altman, Apprey, Caflisch, Cyrus, Davids, Gump, Leary, Levine, Salberg, Stevens, Stoute, Swartz, Suchet, Vaughns, C. White, K. White, Woods). Recent writing on transgenerational trauma has expanded this focus to the sociocultural, creating more space for the interpenetration of the intrapsychic and the sociocultural (e.g., Gonzalez, Grand, Gump, Guralnik, Harris, Hartman, Powell, Rozmarin, Salberg, Sheehi, Stephens, Stevens, Stoute, Vaughans, C. White, K. White).

In her book, *Out of the Sun: On Race and Storytelling*, Esi Edugyan (2021) explores what it means to be seen, and who remains unseen. She writes, "We must first acknowledge the vastly unequal places from which we each speak, the ways some have been denied voices when others are so easily heard."

The subtitle for Danticat's book, *Create Dangerously* is: *The Immigrant Artist at Work*. Creating dangerously, for Danticat, an immigrant from Haiti, alludes to her country's history of violence and political oppression, particularly for artists, intellectuals, and political dissidents. Danticat describes the dysregulating, dissociative impact of sociopolitical, migratory, and relational trauma, and its impact on the creative process.

Importantly, Danticat also highlights a legacy of resilience and survival and tells stories of artists who create despite (or because of) the horrors that drove them from their homelands. As Grand (2018) suggests, "Embedded in catastrophic history, there are manifestations of resourcefulness, dignity, integrity, and compassion" (p. 97). As therapists, in the witnessing of trauma, it is crucial that we "*recognize strengths as well as wounds* ... If we fail to witness horror, we fall prey to its reproduction. If we fail to witness dignity, we reproduce survivors' degradation" (p. 98). I will come back to this essential issue of recognizing and valuing strengths and resilience in the next section.

Psychoanalysis and Disability: Stories Matter

While there has been a relatively recent and long overdue focus on issues of race, class, gender, and intersectionality in psychoanalysis, disability remains an area in which psychoanalysis has been shamefully silent, with a dearth of papers or books addressing disability studies. A recent exception comes to mind: Christina Emanuel's (2022) paper, A white and nondisabled analyst: Owning racism and ableism in the clinical process, in which she "contributes to the project of unsilencing and rendering visible the vicissitudes of ableism and disability" (p. 182). And Ogden ends his paper, "Ontological psychoanalysis or what do you want to be when you grow up?" with a moving case about a patient with cerebral palsy who comes, in the course of analysis, to embrace and "accept himself for who he was in a loving way" (p. 681). This clinical vignette highlights Ogden's central point about the shift to an ontological model focused on being and becoming.

A talented supervisee of mine, who identifies as a therapist with a disability, introduced me to Eli Clare's (2017) book, *Brilliant Imperfection: Grappling with Cure*, which we are reading and reflecting on together. It is an exquisite, intellectually rigorous and wildly original book that weaves race, class, sexuality, gender, and disability, poetry, prose, and politics together, and challenges our deeply held beliefs about the nature of disability and cure. Clare writes:

> Brilliant imperfection is rooted in the nonnegotiable value of body-mind difference. It resists the pressures of normal and abnormal. It defies the easy splitting of natural from unnatural. It has emerged from collective understandings and stubborn survivals. It is expressed in different ways by different communities ... Come sit with me. Let this mosaic that began in conversation spark a hundred new conversations. (xvii)

While not a psychoanalytic text, per se, *Brilliant Imperfection* challenges our fundamental, categorical assumptions about normativity, health and illness, ability and disability, and the vital importance, the fundamental importance, of the stories we tell.

Reading *Brilliant Imperfection* brought to mind the impact of an experience I had back in college at Brown University on my ideology and sense of self as a future therapist working at a school with children with cerebral palsy and spina bifida, and the disdain and disavowal by my psychology professor of my transformative, mind-expanding experience. Most of the children at Meeting Street School were paraplegic or quadriplegic, many unable to speak or move independently. I remember coming back to my dorm room afterward, and collapsing, feeling emotionally and physically exhausted. I think as an able-bodied, athletic person, engaging intimately with children who did not have the freedom of movement of their bodies or the capacity to communicate in words that I had always taken for granted was wrenching, and I dissociated after each visit with them. Yet what stayed with me most powerfully was this school's philosophy, the emphasis on finding and building on children's strengths, capacities, and resilience, helping them to learn and communicate in imaginative, innovative ways.

With all this in mind, I approached my child psychology professor, who researched mother-infant communication, who had agreed to be my advisor for the internship. I said, "Dr. E, I've had this powerful experience at Meeting Street School, but I'm struggling with how to integrate the meaningful experience I've had with the theoretical research and reading I've been doing." He responded, "I don't give a damn about your personal experience. I want a theoretical paper based on research." I was stunned. And furious. I said, "I'm not leaving out my personal experience and the stories of these children. I didn't have to do this internship to write that paper."

This internship and my professor's effort to silence these children's marginalized voices was both infuriating and pivotal for me, a seminal moment in the nascent stages of my education, and later in my writing and in my practice. What all too often gets left out of the teaching of psychology, and psychoanalysis, the essential importance of stories and storytelling, the irreducible subjectivity of each individual and the power, worth, and inclusion of each person's story. Further, though I did not conceptualize it in these terms at 21 years old, the impact on me of working with children who were significantly disabled was a precursor to my thoughts on mutual vulnerability, and a focus on trauma, creativity, and resilience in my writing and approach to psychoanalysis, inhabiting the liminal realm of the imaginations of patient and analyst.

My psychoanalytic ethos also has early roots in my doctoral dissertation on the intergenerational transmission of attachment and trauma across three generations in marginalized families of adolescent mothers. In my dissertation and in subsequent articles from my interview and videotape data, I explored both the continuities and discontinuities of attachment and trauma, focusing especially on essential factors that enabled some young women to break the transgenerational cycle of violence and maltreatment they experienced. Their journeys often entailed disentangling multiple harrowing narratives of psychic ruptures, and reflecting on and processing their complex trauma, in order to establish secure relationships with their babies.

Psychoanalysis and Creativity

Stories about psychoanalysis and creativity also interweave through these chapters, as I explore aspects of creativity as an essential aspect of aliveness and authenticity, and as transformative, emergent in the clinical process. I am thinking here about creativity both in artistic realms and from a broad Winnicottian/Bionian perspective, developed further by Benjamin, Ghent, and Ogden, as an essential aspect of aliveness and authenticity. I believe the capacity to face destructiveness and facilitate mourning are aspects of creativity in the context of human growth. I also want to pick up here on Mitchell's (1993) point about this Winnicottian idea of the importance of the analyst's "surviving the destructiveness of the patient's dread and despair without withdrawing" as a critical aspect of creativity and growth in analysis. Bion (1970) suggests that change is a moment of catastrophe, and that grappling with catastrophic change is an indispensable aspect of psychic growth and creative transformation. This also has resonance in Ogden's (2009) ideas on writing and reading as active, imaginal, relational processes, so that each time you read a text, you're re-writing it in your own voice, bringing a unique perspective and aesthetic to the writing.

I also consider the implications and relevance of psychoanalysis to art and culture, and utilize film, dance, poetry, and literature as creative frames to explore aspects of psychoanalytic process. Transforming ghosts that haunt us into ancestors we can mourn (Atlas, Gump, Harris et al.; Loewald, Powell) and creating new, generative, internal dialogues is one of the challenges inherent in facilitating the creative process. The ghosts of transgenerational trauma linger, reverberating and echoing, creating a sense of après-coup. Finding an authentic, creative voice through the analytic process entails an inhabiting of loss and destruction, disrupting traumatic cycles in order to transform trauma through mourning, creating transitional space for an awakening of desire and creativity.

Transformative Resonance Across Relational, Creative, and Sociocultural Realms

In trying to decide on the order of the chapters in my book, I reflected on the trajectory of my writing and my clinical sensibility over the last 15 years. It's taken me years to directly acknowledge the ways in which I have benefited from White privilege, and grapple with the moral imperative of being implicated in oppressive systems of White supremacy. Over time, as I have come into leadership positions at analytic institutes and as a Joint Editor in-Chief of *Psychoanalytic Dialogues*, I have felt the responsibility, urgency, and empowerment to prioritize anti-racism efforts, to address inequities and injustices in our analytic spaces. The focus of my writing has expanded from the relational and dyadic to the impact of the intersectional and the sociocultural, and the ways in which our multiple identities intersect with our patients.

In the early chapters, I describe transformations across multiple relational realms, including that of analyst and patient, supervisor and supervisee, parent and child. I interrogate the crucial importance of bearing witness, interrogating the challenges, impasses and enactments – the obstacles to, and facilitating of, change and growth. Several of the earlier chapters in the book describe the impact of trauma, creativity, and mutual vulnerability on memory, agency, and aliveness, and build on notions of creativity as transformative, emergent in the clinical process.

Moving further into the impact of the sociocultural on the psyche and on clinical process, later chapters focus on the challenge of staying enlivened when locked in an endless present through rape, psychic trauma, and incarceration, the impact of intergenerational and migration trauma on creating one's own story, and the *moral injury* at the heart of our nation's history, the ways in which we're all "implicated" in the iniquitous history of our nation, as *beneficiaries or descendants* (Rothberg, 2019). This entails facing ways in which White Americans have benefited from the institutionalization of White privilege and control. It demands of all of us a sense of responsibility, and an obligation to participate in the dismantling of racism, in the deconstructing and reconstruction of more equitable, anti-racist analytic spaces.

In Chapter One, "Transformative Resonance Across Relational Realms," I explore ways in which, as psychoanalysts, our own relational stories, our "wounds that must serve as tools" (Harris, 2009), represent both our greatest liabilities and potential for change, at times facilitating and at times impeding our capacity to engage deeply in the analytic process. Building on writings by Aron, Bass, Benjamin, Bromberg, Davies, Ehrenberg, Ghent, and Harris, I explore the complexity of impasse and resonance across various relational realms and consider ways in which our patients' growth and the healing of old wounds is intimately connected to the analyst's openness to her own vulnerabilities.

I describe how a profound piece of work in my personal analysis around healing in my relationship with my then young son resonated in my work with a long-term patient, enlivening and deepening the treatment. I reflect on how I drew on the interpenetrating experiences of analyst, patient, mother, and child; how transformative experiences in my own analysis and subsequently, in my relationship with my son, opened potential space in my work with a patient, and in her relationship with her own son, making possible a deeper level of vulnerability, intimacy, and mutual recognition (Levine, 2009).

In Chapter Two, "Into Thin Air: The Interweaving of Shame, Recognition, and Creativity," I examine ways in which shame, recognition, and creativity are coconstructed in an analytic process. Focusing on my work with Julia, an artist who was extraordinarily creative in her dreams, metaphors, and artistic vision, yet spent much of her life struggling to make art, I consider both conscious and unconscious factors that open or close down vitality and intimacy in our work with patients, and the importance of spontaneity and risk taking, particularly in negotiating impasses in treatment.

I explore how patients' access to their imagination, dreams, and other unconscious realms may be intimately connected to the analyst's variable and shifting receptivity to her own imagination and creativity and consider the ways in which creativity is both solitary and co-constructed. I contemplate ways in which shame and recognition interpenetrate with creativity, both within psychoanalysis and within the artistic process (Levine, 2012). My patient, Julia, an artist who struggled mightily with creative blocks, and I went through phases in the therapy in which there was a shared sense of vivacity, a creative sense of "flow," in which she imagined art projects she wanted to make. But inevitably, the aliveness would disappear, as if into thin air, and she would shift into a more discouraged state, in which her art felt far away and inaccessible.

I also reflect on Julia's reaction to reading the paper, as someone who struggled throughout her life with feeling invisible and unheard, the impact of seeing herself reflected through my eyes, how surprised and moved she was by the impact she had had on me. This was a powerful intersubjective process in and of itself, adding another layer of resonance across relational realms. She said, "I had no idea what I expected. It's a story—my story—and you and I are the main characters."

In Chapter Three, "Surviving Destruction and Its Creative Potential for Agency and Desire," I examine ways in which the courage to engage deeply in psychoanalysis entails struggling to free ourselves from old identifications and constraints (Levine, 2016a), and taking the risk of accompanying our patients into the abyss, so that they are no longer alone there with their anguish. Then their pain can become shareable and bearable, decreasing their sense of shame. I discuss the importance of recognizing and mobilizing our own capacity for destructiveness and agency, of mourning un-grieved losses in order to have the courage to swim together in dangerous, deadly waters. I investigate ways in which a mutual survival of a suicidal patient's destructiveness opened potential space for creativity, agency, and desire in both of us.

Barely six months into our work together, Jack rode his bicycle up to the George Washington Bridge and climbed the fence, intending to jump, then re-considered. I felt pushed to the precipice myself, to the edge of my capacity as an analyst, as Jack got deeply into my psyche, under my skin, kept me up at night when he was suicidal. I believe my struggling to hang in there with him in the face of his deadness and deadliness, without retaliating or withdrawing helped us both imagine a sense of agency, psychic future (Loewald, 1960; Cooper, 2016b) and creative possibility.

In Chapter Four, "Mutual Vulnerability: Destruction and Reparation," I explore the creative potential, as well as the profound challenges, of mutual vulnerability in psychoanalysis, building on Ferenczi, Aron, Bass, Benjamin, Davies, and Ehrenberg's efforts to open the analytic field to the intersubjectivity of both analyst and patient, and the dialogue of unconsciouses, while maintaining the crucial asymmetry of the analytic relationship (Aron, 1996). Mutual vulnerability entails a willingness to be deeply unsettled and dysregulated by our most wounded patients. In my patient, Lisa's fierce determination to come into being, and in our mutual efforts to survive each other's ruthlessness (Winnicott, 1969) and attacks on linking (Bion, 1959), we each struggle to recognize and own malignant 'not-me' versions of ourselves (Bromberg, 1998), as we reach toward reparation, mutual recognition, and healing (Levine, 2016b).

Ferro (2006), building on Bion, suggested that the analyst constantly receives, metabolizes, and transforms the patient's verbal and non-verbal stimuli into ongoing reverie and that the patient's and analyst's psychic collisions create a bipersonal analytic field (Baranger and Baranger, 2008) that is perpetually dreamed and re-dreamed. Building on Bleger's and the Barrangers' notions of the analytic setting as a dynamic field which includes elements of the frame, and aspects of time and space, I also discuss the intersecting of two subjectivities and psychoanalytic histories. I illustrate how aspects of our personal analysis, supervision, past and current experiences with other patients reside, often unconsciously or preconsciously, in the analyst, emerging unbidden in reveries, dreams, and associations, and creating unanticipated opportunities—or enactments—in our work with patient (Levine, 2009).

In Chapter Five, "Pina Bausch: Trauma, Memory, and Creative Transformation," I use Pina Bausch's dance as a creative frame to explore the ways in which creativity in psychoanalysis can serve as a vital window into different registers of time and traumatic loss, transforming trauma through mourning, and creating the potential for a reawakening of aliveness and desire in both analyst and patient. In the extraordinary documentary *Pina* (2011), Wim Wenders's homage to Pina Bausch, dancers collide and fall in unexpected ways. They slip! and fall backward or sideways, suspended momentarily in midair before being caught by another dancer at the last possible moment. Past and future collapse as the powerful 3D filming brings us, the audience, right into the intensity of the present. And time falls away. It's violent, erotic, immersive. The film holds multiple layers of trauma and creativity, trauma interrupting/disrupting creativity and time, and then creativity reimagined, re-enlivened, and co-created as transitional object.

In this chapter, I focus on the intersection of trauma, creativity, and mourning and build on Steven Cooper's recent work on the centrality of mourning in moving from dissociation to aliveness, creativity, and the capacity to play in analysis. I describe my work with another artist patient who is desperate to leave his past behind, to heal from his early trauma of fear and abandonment, but his body keeps him trapped in the past, with wordless emotions and feelings and nameless dread. Like Pina Bausch's dancers, struggling to bear trauma, to wake from the fog of dissociation, to break free from the ties that bind them. While there is a powerful longing to connect, to embrace and be embraced, there's trepidation, vulnerability, visible, and invisible barriers to connecting.

In Chapter Six, "Finding Creative Means of Staying Enlivened when Locked in an Endless Present: Deconstructing the film, Room" I read the heart-wrenching film, *Room* from multiple, overlapping perspectives. I explore the human capacity for resilience in the face of unspeakable trauma, and its implications for psychoanalysis, drawing on the seminal work of Viktor Frankl, Sam Gerson, and Robert Jay Lifton on the vital importance of witnessing and meaning-making. In the film, an adolescent girl named Joy, is abducted, imprisoned, and impregnated by her captor. Though her son, Jack is the product of rape, Joy is determined to create an imaginative, even joyful world for him within the confines of Room. This desperate imperative, Winnicott's primary maternal preoccupation as a means of survival, enables her to channel the chaos of her ongoing despair into a creative, life-sustaining endeavor.

I also interweave stories from Bryan Stevenson's extraordinary book, *Just Mercy*, about the lives of incarcerated men, women and adolescents he has defended, and the crucial importance of witnessing in restoring human dignity. Stevenson, the founder of the Equal Justice Initiative in Montgomery, Alabama, also writes about the horrors of mass incarceration, as well as the dehumanization and racial inequities of the American criminal justice system. I believe Stevenson's writing has essential implications for psychoanalysis in leaning into individual and collective brokenness and mutual recognition as a source of healing.

In Chapter Seven, "Becoming the Storyteller of One's Own Life," I riff on Rebecca Solnit's (2013) ideas on the faraway nearby, stories as compasses and architecture, a way of traveling from here to there. I investigate the impact of intergenerational and migration trauma on aliveness, temporality and intersubjectivity, and on what Seligman (2016) calls, becoming "a self in time." I describe my work with Darya, a Lebanese American woman whose vitality and aliveness were crushed by the weight of dissociated, unspoken racial melancholia (Eng and Han, 2000).

As a child, Darya had been a storyteller with a wondrous imagination, who dreamed of becoming a writer, or an artist. But when she first came to see me, at 25, she was overwhelmed by a profound existential dread, tormented by frequent somatic ailments, and a terror that she was dying. I felt as if she were carrying the weight of history, the anguish of past generations in her body, as if there were ghosts hovering, holding her body and mind captive and that I would need to get to know those ghosts intimately, over time. I wondered whether Darya's paralysis was a form of melancholic sacrifice (Eng and Han, 2000), as each time she gained some traction, each time she experienced a sense of agency and intentionality, each time she was inspired by an act of imagination, there was a collapse, an act of destruction that thwarted any forward movement or creative growth.

I began writing the eighth and final chapter in the spring of 2020 during a cataclysmic collision of the COVID-19 pandemic and a long overdue, White awakening, and subsequent racist backlash to the pandemic of anti-Black racism, police violence, and racial trauma. This reckoning with the structural and institutional racism embedded in American history, culture, and politics was triggered by the murder of George Floyd, a Black man by Derek Chauvin, a White Minneapolis cop, one of innumerable killings of innocent Black men.

In this chapter, through clinical encounters as a White analyst working with several women of color, I argue for a radical shift in our conception of the analytic frame, necessitating stepping outside of a familiar, comfortable role in which we have been taught to follow what patients bring to analysis. Rather than waiting for our patients to bring up issues of race, I believe it behooves White analysts to take the lead in listening for and speaking directly about race, racism, and racial identity, to make it clear that we are invested in, and up for these challenging discussions.

I contend that as psychoanalysts, we must step into our discomfort, wrestle with our shame and shared vulnerability, and the ways in which we are all implicated; not equally, but meaningfully. I emphasize the crucial imperative for White analysts of struggling with our inclination toward silence, complicity, and dissociation. Clearly this requires sensitivity, care, deep listening, and a willingness to step into discomfort, make mistakes, try to repair racialized enactments when they inevitably occur, and, as Kirkland Vaughans (2022) suggests, in his discussion of my paper in *Psychoanalytic*

Dialogues (Levine, 2022), to "reach *out* rather than *down*, to construct necessary scaffolding to bridge the divide in cross-racial dyads." In her discussion, Adrienne Harris (2022) writes,

> The patient is given the freedom to say what comes to mind but this could effectively be a screen behind which the White analyst hides. Given the gravitas of matters of race and empowerment and privilege, where is the analyst's moral obligation to name the unspoken ghosts and living trauma agents, alive in the clinical setting?

And finally, Michelle Stephens (2022) queries:

> The deeper implication Lauren Levine finds herself wrestling with in her consulting room, especially with her patients of color, is, what does it mean to think about relational racialization as a process that we are all subject to and subjected by, even if with more or less detrimental, corrosive effects on our senses of self?

In this final chapter, I reflect on issues of power, grief, and rage, holding in mind both "unbridgeable gaps in racialized experience, the (im)possibilities of resolution regarding racial alienation and re-cognition, as well as possibilities for accompaniment and generativity in working clinically with racialized trauma" (Stevens, 2020). I explore ways in which White supremacy affects—*and infects*—all of us, in our bodies, in our histories, and in the stories we tell, and pass down to our children and grandchildren.

We are currently in the midst of a terrifying sociopolitical backlash by the radical right to suppress our stories, to silence and whitewash the white supremacy and racism embedded in our history and culture. We must face our legacy of chattel slavery and the slaughter of Indigenous people on which our country was founded and fight the enactment of laws dictating the teaching of a false narrative of history, banning books and free speech about race, gender, and sexuality, banning abortion and threats of overturning laws on same-sex relationships and marriage, and contraception access. What would it take to bear witness to our collective sins instead of denying the history in which we are all implicated (Rothberg, McKay and Mark,

2022) not equally, but meaningfully, as perpetrators, victims, or their descendants or ancestors?

The power to share our stories with a listening, witnessing other is foundational. As analysts, this requires courage to swim together in dangerous waters, to go to the depths, to take the risk of accompanying our patients into the abyss. Then they are no longer alone there with their anguish, as their pain can become shareable and bearable, decreasing their sense of shame (Levine, 2016a). But as psychoanalysis also entails dangerous undertakings for us as analysts, we need to create life rafts in our work (Pass, 2019), to keep us afloat as we absorb and are penetrated by shards of previously unbearable trauma (Corbett, 2012; Harris, 2009).

I have been deeply inspired by Bryan Stevenson, civil rights attorney, author of *Just Mercy,* and founder of the Equal Justice Initiative. In *Just Mercy* (2014), Stevenson traces the insidious legacy of slavery, racial violence, and trauma embedded in American history and their impact on the vast racial inequities of mass incarceration. He tells stories of trauma, survival, and resilience, emphasizing the crucial importance of witnessing and storytelling in restoring human dignity. Stevenson describes the ubiquity of brokenness and the essential importance of witnessing. He writes:

> We are all broken by something. We all share the condition of brokenness even if our brokenness is not equivalent. However, our brokenness is also the source of our common humanity, the basis for our shared search for comfort, meaning, and healing. Our shared vulnerability and our imperfection nurtures and sustains our capacity for compassion. (p. 289)

I will end by adding one more voice to this conversation on transformative resonance and psychoanalysis as creating dangerously. The remarkable feminist writer, philosopher, and cultural critic, Bell Hooks writes about the ubiquity of fear, particularly racialized fear, and the importance of love. It feels deeply relevant to the relational psychoanalytic project, as well as how we find ways to connect across difference and live together on this fragile planet of ours. In *All about Love*, Hooks (2001) writes:

In our society we make much of love and say little about fear. Yet we are all terribly afraid most of the time … Fear is the primary force upholding structures of domination. It promotes the desire for separation, the desire not to be known. When we are taught that safety lies always with sameness, then difference, of any kind, will appear as a threat. When we choose to love, we choose to move against fear, against alienation and separation. The choice to love is a choice to connect, to find ourselves in the other. (p. 93)

I/We, You/Us, Just Us[*]

References

Abraham, N. (1988). Notes on the phantom: A complement to Freud's metapsychology. *Critical Inquiry*, 13: 287–292.

Abraham, N. and Torok, M. (1984). "The lost object—Me": Notes on identification within the crypt. *Psychoanalytic Inquiry*, 4, 221–242.

Aron, L. (1996). *A meeting of minds: Mutuality in psychanalysis*. Hillsdale, NJ: The Analytic Press.

Aron, L. and Atlas, G. (2015). Dialogues paper.

Atlas, G. (2022). *Emotional inheritance: A therapist, her patients, and the legacy of trauma*. New York: Little, Brown.

Baranger, M. and Baranger, W. (2008). The analytic situation as a dynamic field. *The International Journal of Psychoanalysis*, 89: 795–826.

Bass, A. (2015). The Dialogue of Unconsciouses: Mutual Analysis and the Uses of the Self in Contemporary Relational Psychoanalysis. *Psychoanalytic Dialogues*, 25(1): 2–17.

Bion, W. (1991). Memories from the future.

Bion, W. (1970). Change as a moment of catastrophe.

Bion, W. (1959). Attacks on linking. *International Journal of Psychoanalysis*, 40: 308–315.

Bromberg, P. (2006). Potholes on the royal road: Or is it an abyss? In *Awakening the Dreamer: Clinical journeys*. London: Routledge.

Bromberg, P. (1998). Standing in the spaces: The multiplicity of self and the psychoanalytic relationship. Book Page 511.

Clare, E. (2017). *Brilliant imperfection: Grappling with cure*. Durham: Duke University Press.

[*] Claudia Rankine, Just Us: An American Conversation (2020).

Cooper, S.H. (2016a). *The melancholic errand of psychoanalysis: Exploring the analyst's relationship to the depressive position*. London, UK: Routledge.

Cooper, S.H. (2016b). Mourning, regeneration, and the psychic future: A discussion of Levine's "A mutual survival of destructiveness and its creative potential for agency and desire". *Psychoanalytic Dialogues*, 26: 56–62.

Corbett, K. (2012). All of these things will happen. Graduation Speech at NYU Postdoctoral Program in Psychotherapy and psychoanalysis, New York, NY.

Danticat, E. (2011). *Create dangerously: The immigrant artist at work*. New York: Vintage Books.

Dowd, D. (2018). The unfreezing of time in the haunted hours. *Psychoanalytic Dialogues*, 28: 69–77.

Dufourmantelle, A. (2019). *In praise of risk*. New York: Fordham University Press.

Edugyan, E. (2021). *Out of the sun: On race and storytelli*ng. Canada: House of Anansi Press.

Emanuel, C. (2022). A white and nondisabled analyst: Owning racism and ableism in the clinical process. *Psychoanalysis, Self and Context*, 17: 181–195.

Eng, D. and Han (2000). A dialogue on racial melancholia. *Psychoanalytic Dialogues*, 10: 667–700.

Faimberg, H. (2005). *The telescoping of generations: Listening to the narcissistic links between generations*. London: Routledge.

Ferro, A. (2006). Trauma, reverie and the field. *The Psychoanalytic Quarterly*, 75: 1045–1056.

Ghent, E. (1990). Masochism, submission, surrender: Masochism as a perversion of surrender. *Contemporary Psychoanalysis*, 26: 108–136.

Grand, S. (2018). The other within: White shame and Native American genocide. *Contemporary Psychoanalysis*, 54: 84–102.

Harris, A. (2022). Encountering shame with stamina in clinical work with race and racism. *Psychoanalytic Dialogues*, 32: 121–125.

Harris (2009). You must remember this. *Psychoanalytic Dialogues*, 19: 2–21.

Harris, A. (2010). The Analyst's Omnipotence and the Analyst's Melancholy.

Hooks, B. (2001). *All about love: New visions*. New York: William Morrow.

Laub, D. (2017). Reestablishing the internal "Thou" in testimony of trauma. In J. Alpert and E. Goren (Eds.) *Psychoanalysis, trauma, and community: History and contemporary reappraisals*. London: Routledge.

Layton, L. (2019). Transgenerational hauntings: Toward a social psycho-analysis and an ethic of dis-illusionment. *Psychoanalytic Dialogues*, 29: 105–121.

Levine, L. (2009). Transformative aspects of our own analysesand their resonance in our work with our patients. *Psychoanalytic Dialogue*, 19: 454–462.

Levine, L. (2012). Into thin air: The co-construction of shame, recognition and creativity in an analytic process. *Psychoanalytic Dialogues*, 22: 456–471.

Levine, L. (2016a). A mutual survival of destructiveness and its creative potential for agency and desire. *Psychoanalytic Dialogues*, 26: 36–49.

Levine, L. (2016b). Mutual vulnerability: Intimacy, psychic collisionsand the shards of trauma. *Psychoanalytic Dialogues*, 26: 571–579.

Mendelsohn, S. (2018). Poetics in the clinical encounter. *Psychoanalytic Dialogues*, 28: 78–85.

Mitchell, S. (1993). *Hope and dread in psychoanalysis*. New York: Basic Books.

Ogden, T. (2019). Ontological psychoanalysis or "What do you want to be when you grow up?" *Psychoanalytic Quarterly*, 88: 661–684.

Ogden, T. (2009). *Rediscovering psychoanalysis: Thinking and dreaming, learning and forgetting*. London: Routledge.

Pass, S. (2019). Tyler in the Labyrinth: A Young Child's Journey from Chaos to Coherence. *Psychoanalytic Dialogues*, 29: 594–609.

Powell, D. (2018). Race, African Americans and psychoanalysis: Collective silence in the therapeutic conversation. *JAPA*, 66: 1021–1049.

Rankine, C. (2020). *Just us: An American conversation*. Minneapolis: Graywolf Press.

Rothberg, M. (2019). *The implicated subject: Beyond victims and perpe-trators*. Stanford CA: Stanford University Press.

Salberg, J. (2017). The texture of traumatic attachment: Presence and ghostly absence in transgenerational transmission. In J. Salberg and S. Grand, (Eds.) *Wounds of history: Repair and resilience in the transge-nerational transmission of trauma*. London: Routledge.

Schwartz Cooney, A. (2021). *Vitalization in psychoanalysis: Perspectives on being and becoming*. London: Routledge.

Seligman, S. (2016). Disorders of temporality and the subjective experience of time: Unresponsive objects and the vacuity of the future. *Psychoanalytic Dialogues*, 26: 110–128.

Solnit, R. (2013). *The faraway nearby*. New York: Penguin.

Stephens, M. (2022). Relational Racialization and segregated whiteness. *Psychoanalytic Dialogues*, 32: 114–120.

Stevens, G. (2020). Racial alienation, the (im)possibilities of resolution, and the absent/present other. *Psychoanalytic Dialogues*, 30: 716–722.

Stevenson, B. (2014). *Just mercy:* A story of justice and redemption. New York: Random House.

Vaughans, K. (2022). Commentary on Lauren Levine's Interrogating race, shame and mutual vulnerability. *Psychoanalytic Dialogues*, 32: 126–129.

Winnicott, D. W. (1969). The use of an object. *International Journal of Psychoanalysis*, 50: 711–716.

Chapter 1

Transformative Resonance Across Relational Realms

In this chapter, I will explore the complexity of impasse and resonance across multiple relational realms and consider ways in which our patients' stories and the healing of old wounds are intimately connected to the analyst's openness to her own vulnerabilities and ungrieved losses (Harris, 2009; Levine, 2009; Levine, 2016a). I will describe how a powerful piece of work in my own analysis around the struggle to connect with my young son in the face of his impulsivity and aggression resonated in my work with a patient, Susan, and subsequently created new possibilities in her relationship with her teenage son. Though I had never talked with Susan about my son, I believe that on an implicit relational level (Stern et al., 1998), the experiences in my own analysis and healing in my relationship with my son both created barriers and opened potential space with my patient, enlivening and deepening the treatment. In the process, Susan discovered new places within herself, which enabled her to "join" her son in ways she had never thought possible.

While psychoanalysis has embraced relational notions of intersubjectivity and mutuality in the realm of countertransference, less is known about what Harris (2009) calls "the analyst's wounds that must serve as tools, aspects of the analyst's capacities that are simultaneously brakes and potentials for change." Our own relational, sociocultural, and intergenerational history at times facilitates, and at other times hinders our capacity to engage deeply in the analytic process (Atlas, 2022; Gump, 2010; Harris, 2009; Kuchuck, 2014). Aspects of our personal analysis reside, often unconsciously or

DOI: 10.4324/9781003367475-2

preconsciously in the analyst, creating unexpected obstacles and opportunities in our work with our patients.

Years ago, the mother of a young child patient told me the following story. Tired and cranky after a wonderful, but very long day in the park, her little boy's behavior escalated into a full-blown tantrum. Kicking and screaming, at some point, he picked up a belt and hit her—with the metal end. After taking a deep breath, the mother gently put her arms around him and they sank down to the floor together and he began to cry, finally allowing her to comfort him. Blown away by this mother's capacity to respond lovingly in the face of her son's aggression, I asked her, "How were you able to do that?" She responded, "Someone very wise once told me, that when your kid is at his *worst,* he needs you the *most.*"

That story has stayed with me for 20 years. It still brings tears to my eyes. I find it deceptively simple and surprisingly profound, because in reality, when your kid is at his worst, particularly in an ongoing, challenging way, it can bring out the worst in you as a parent. To have the grace and fortitude to take a step back and reflect, to take a deep breath and allow your rage to dissipate, to be able to tune into your out- of-control child's underlying need for holding and soothing rather than reacting to his bad behavior; that is an inspired act, and something to aspire to. The story also highlights ways in which our patients' fault lines and vulnerabilities can, at times, collide with our own in surprising, unpredictable ways (Levine, 2016b). But I'm getting ahead of myself.

At age four, my son was hyperactive and impulsive, with expressive and receptive language processing issues. Frustrated by his difficulty communicating and being understood, he was often aggressive at home and in trouble at school. This was many years ago, but I can still remember him standing in the school yard, fists clenched, tears streaming down his face, yelling at another child who was running away from him, "You're not listening to me!" It broke my heart. I was desperate to help him. I was his staunch advocate and supporter. But, privately I also felt frustrated, angry, and helpless, as we were often stuck in polarizing power struggles.

In her paper, "'Betwixt the Dark and the Daylight' of Maternal Subjectivity," Kraemer (1996) deconstructs romanticized, idealized notions of the "good enough" mother, and explores the complexity and anguish of maternal anger, shame, and helplessness. I would argue that the idealization of motherhood in our culture creates an even greater burden for mothers in our profession. It felt particularly painful to me that I seemed to be able to help other families in my practice wrestling with similar issues, yet I could not unlock the secret of how to reach my own son. What would my patients think if they knew how much I was struggling with my son? I felt enormous shame in "not knowing" how to calm him, heal him. It wasn't that I did not see the sweetness in him, the passion and exuberance; we had many affectionate, loving moments. It just felt so hard to "hold" him in a Winnicottian sense, to stay connected in an ongoing way in the face of his provocative behavior.

Although he was receiving a range of therapies, I believe it was a challenging piece of work in my own analysis that had the greatest impact. Having grown up in a family of girls, the oldest, responsible "together" child, I experienced this intense boy as "unknowable" on some level, hard to identify with. Feeling overwhelmed and exhausted, it was difficult for me to acknowledge that what he might need was *more* of me, but *something different* that I had not been able to give him before. My son was struggling mightily at school and at home, acting aggressively in ways that frightened other children, and as much I was trying to help him, it was not making enough of a difference, and things were escalating. So, I struggled with my analyst to own my part in it, determined to be there for my son in the ways he needed me to be. My analyst challenged me to see what I had been missing, to understand my son's aggression not only as biologically driven, but as a protest, as a response to being misunderstood. I began to see how difficult it was for me to feel "in sync" with him when he was agitated or acting out, that I was responding more "from the outside" by trying to contain him. I began to realize the importance of not just reacting to his behavior, which was making me anxious or angry, or both, but rather trying to stay calm, to join him from the inside. Gradually, his agitated states began to feel less foreign to me, and he began to feel less "bad" and more understood.

How did this happen? It took time for me to recognize the degree of anguish that my son and I were both in, and to acknowledge that we needed help. It felt shameful to reveal to my analyst the extent of the difficulties in my relationship with my son. I worried that she would be critical, or see me as a bad mother. Although we had never talked directly about her grown children, I had the idealized fantasy that she was a wonderful mother, deeply committed to her children, that she had weathered challenging moments herself, and that she drew on her experiences of mothering in our work together. Unconsciously, I think I was terrified of recognizing and owning my own aggression and destructiveness. But it was through my beginning to acknowledge the extent of my frustration and anger at my son that I became more able to empathize with him. As my analyst helped me get to know and give voice to those buried, shameful parts of myself, I began to see the path to reaching my son.

Without ever meeting him, somehow my analyst had faith in him, and I suppose, in me as well. She saw his sensitivity and vulnerability, his capacity to be healed and held, through me. Even when I couldn't yet, even when I felt desperate, frustrated, not "getting" him, she believed he would be all right, and helped me to believe it, to feel that whoever he was, was "good enough." She helped me to see the dis-avowed pain that lay underneath, fueling his provocative behavior, the pain of rejection by other children, the pain of not feeling un-derstood on multiple levels. And when he felt known, recognized and loved for all of him, he settled down, his aggression *began to fall away.* My son's attentional and language difficulties had clearly compromised his ability to regulate his emotional experience, but as I became more able to join him and help him put his experience into words, he calmed down. I could feel and see the impact it was having on him, on his sense of self as well as on his behavior. It became ap-parent over time just how sensitive and articulate he could be about his own emotional experience and attuned to the affective experiences of others.

I want to convey what a unique perspective this was, what a re-velation. Almost everyone was relating to him as a difficult, de-manding child. The feedback he was getting all around him, from many family, friends, and teachers was that his behavior was un-acceptable, that *he* needed to change. So, not surprisingly, he had begun to feel like a "bad boy." Of course, the parallel message to me, as his mother, was to set more limits, to *control* his behavior. We both felt the shame of not being good enough. But what I began to dis-cover was that he needed me to be different from everyone else, to not react to him based solely on his behavior and other peoples' expectations. Like the mother who was able to wrap her arms around her son after he hit her with the belt buckle, to soothe him and help him regulate his distress, to connect to his shame in feeling out of control, I discovered new places within myself that I could draw upon to meet his underlying emotional needs.

There was something initially frightening, but ultimately liberating about letting go in the presence of my analyst, helping me break out of a state of aloneness and collapse, which allowed me to fall apart, to be a mess, to acknowledge the depths of my own pain, anger, and helplessness. Not surprisingly, I began to feel freer to express aggressive feelings toward my analyst as well, to provoke and challenge her directly, and over time, we developed an increasing capacity to play with aggression within the context of the analytic relationship. This led to a greater sense of emotional freedom, authenticity, and aliveness in me, which in turn enabled me to provide that "safe enough" environment for my son, so that I could embrace *all of him*. My son and I were both longing for an experience of "surrender," in Ghent's (1990) words, "a deep yearning to be found and recognized" (p. 132). When it goes well, psychoanalysis gives one the experience of being in a relationship that feels safe enough that one can begin to feel less ashamed and humiliated by, and more aware of those split-off, unacceptable parts of oneself (Harris, 2009). There was something so powerful for me about my analyst's faith in me and in my son, her embracing of our vulnerabilities, and her belief in our resilience and capacity for change. I resonate deeply with Davies' (2003) reflection that:

> It is not only that the patient discovers himself held in the mind of the analyst ... but more significantly, it is *who* the patient discovers residing in his analyst's mind, as well as the *transformation* of that *who*—the multiple and emergent *who's*—that determine the breadth and scope of therapeutic potential. (p. 25)

One Monday morning on the way to school, my son was agitated, distressed, *not* listening. I felt momentarily exasperated, and then I felt something shift in me as I saw him with fresh eyes. I asked, "Is it hard to go back to school on Monday when we've been together all weekend?" He stopped moving and looked me directly in the eye. "Because it's hard for me to go back to work. I miss you when I'm at work." His *whole body calmed down,* and he took my hand and we walked to school together.

Years later, my son, the little boy in the schoolyard who cried out, "You're not listening to me!" has become a musician: guitar player, singer, composer of original music. He has found his voice—and it's passionate and soulful.

Solow Glennon (2007) describes how singing was a source of healing for her in the mourning process after the death of her first husband. She suggests that "access to genuine, heartfelt emotion can be facilitated by artistic expression as well as by the immediate experience of an authentic affective engagement with an other." Drawing on Ogden's (2005) work, she then proposes that at its heart, psychoanalysis seeks to foster authenticity, aliveness, and creativity, which leads me to the second part of my story.

Having never been in therapy, fearful of the ghosts and unbearable affects that would emerge if we delved too deeply into her past, Susan asked in the first session whether we could focus exclusively on helping her leave her emotionally abusive husband, and on her tremendous fears about the impact of divorce on her son. Once I gave her permission to define the boundaries and determine the pace of our work together, Susan felt safe enough to begin treatment. I soon understood that Susan was a woman who had experienced significant trauma, most of it dissociated, and that it would take us a while to get to those darker places.

Over the years, Susan made remarkable strides. She began to separate from and make peace with her domineering father, mobilized herself to leave her marriage, survived breast cancer, and began the process of mourning her mother, who had committed suicide when Susan was four years old. But, even with all the growth and change, there was still a subtle affective flatness, a constriction and caution, and difficulty taking action. Susan periodically asked me if I thought she was making progress, wondering if I was "pushing her enough." Though we explored this, and questions about what blocked her from feeling more spontaneous and empowered, this didn't enliven the treatment in any sustained, meaningful way.

Susan grew up with her father and younger sister in Chicago. As I mentioned, her mother committed suicide when Susan was four. There had been no room for mourning in her family. It was clear that her father, a lawyer, traumatized by the death of his own mother in childhood, could not tolerate the pain of mourning his wife's death or help his young children do so, particularly given the unbearable trauma and guilt of suicide. Thus, there were at least two generations of maternal loss and abandonment, unmetabolized, unprocessed. Rather than helping his children keep memories of their mother alive, he tried to bury all traces of her.

Not surprisingly, Susan had few memories of her mother, and it took time for her to develop a real curiosity about who her mother was, as well as an appreciation of the impact of the loss. Not wanting to anger her volatile father or cause him more pain, Susan had refrained from asking questions about her mother or the exact circumstances of her death, which had been shrouded in mystery. We explored questions about knowing and not knowing, wanting and not wanting to know. Eventually, it dawned on Susan that her mother had never recovered from a severe post-partum depression, or possibly post-partum psychosis after her birth.

Susan had been a good girl, a superior student, eager for her critical father's approval. Susan's maternal grandmother was also a significant parental figure, a gentle, loving presence, the only person who provided unconditional love. She died when Susan was in her early twenties, and Susan married soon afterward. Though she had doubts about her husband, she deferred to his pressure to get married, anxious for the security of a relationship. He was familiar: critical, controlling, and ultimately emotionally abusive. They had one child, a son with significant learning and attentional issues as well as emotional vulnerabilities.

When Susan entered treatment, in her early forties, she was terrified of the impact that divorce would have on her son, as he was already so vulnerable. However, her husband was also emotionally abusive toward her son, and Susan ultimately realized that she needed to move out for her son's sake as well as her own. After a number of years of therapy, and with great trepidation, she left the marriage, only to be diagnosed with breast cancer soon afterward.

After enduring a mastectomy and chemotherapy, facing her own mortality at age 48, and the fear of abandoning her son by dying, Susan fell into an agitated depression. Having always been high functioning and self-sufficient, it was terrifying to her to feel such helplessness and despair. During this period, sessions never felt long enough; it was uncharacteristically difficult for her to leave each one. I felt her maternal longing and hunger in a way I had never experienced before.

Enormously relieved as she was beginning to come out of the depression, she came in one day and told me, out of the blue, that she was planning to move to Chicago to be close to her father, leaving her son to live with her ex-husband in New York City. She rationalized that her son would be able to manage with his father in New York. It so took me by surprise that I almost fall off my chair! Or more accurately, I felt the urge to jump out of my chair and shake her. Are you kidding me?

How to understand this enactment after all the concerns she had had about the impact of divorce on her son, and her anguish about the possibility of abandoning him to his abusive father if she had not survived the cancer? What was she trying to communicate through this enactment that "was not yet otherwise expressible ... a signal of what was stirring just beneath the surface of the waters?" (Jacobs, 1991, p. 49)

I was powerfully aware of the risk of intergenerational repetition of abandonment: her father's mother had died when her father was a child, her own mother had committed suicide when Susan was four, and now Susan was on the verge of abandoning her son to the care of his unstable father. Of course, there was another threat of abandonment lurking just below the surface of our mutual awareness: We were still right in the thick of our work together. Where did she think she was *going?* Suddenly, I was thrust into the position of the little girl being left without warning. What was Susan trying to help me understand about her experience that I had not been aware of before? Bass (2003) has suggested that in enactments, the analyst is especially challenged to locate in herself personal forms of creative responsiveness to the complex subtleties of an analytic moment, and the fate of the analytic process itself often hinges on the patient's and the analyst's both coming to new, expanded modes of self-awareness. (p. 661)

While offering Susan my interpretation about the repetition of intergenerational abandonment was critical, I think that what really allowed us to begin to think, to reflect together on this enactment, was that it resonated powerfully for me, and I drew on my experience, as a mother who had had to reckon with the ways in which I had abandoned my own son, perhaps in more subtle, but still powerful ways. I struggled to lean into my own experience with my son, to tap into the challenges of embracing a child who has hit you with a belt, the metal end. Shifting back and forth between the positions of mother and child, trying to hold *the relationship in mind,* I struggled to create a transitional space of thirdness (Benjamin, 2004) in order to get some greater perspective on this enactment.

I felt an urgency to break through Susan's denial of the devastating impact this would have on her son, while being mindful of not shaming *her.* As I wrote in a previous paper, "shame can travel insidiously across relational realms, passed back and forth, alternately projected and introjected, from analyst to patient" and back again (Levine, 2012). Susan, like me, had been a very different child from her son and she too found it difficult to identify with, and to join with her son. Initially, I had not seen the degree to which she was emotionally abandoning him, because of my own identification with her as a good mother doing the best she could, a good girl with a challenging boy. Clearly, identifications with patients, overlaps in our lives and histories, can present potential blind spots as well as "bright spots," or opportunities for resonance (Goldberger, 1993). But the threat of this multigenerational abandonment broke through our mutual dissociation so that we could begin to understand how her unconscious identification with her mother had led to the threat of this intergenerational repetition of abandonment.

For the first time, Susan began to grapple directly with her mother's death as a suicide and the treatment took on an affective urgency that we had never experienced together. As we processed this enactment together, Susan gained access to deep layers of unconscious identification with her mother, and we began to understand her depression and the repetition of abandonment as an unconscious attempt to *get to know* her mother, to *feel* her through this experience, from the inside out. Having hit bottom in this depression, she began to understand for the first time, the depths of her mother's anguish before she killed herself—by jumping off a building. She could finally empathize with how excruciating it had been for her mother to feel so hopeless. This allowed her to become conscious of her anger at her mother for abandoning her, to access the rage and guilt underlying the sadness of the loss. Susan had looked down into the abyss but hadn't jumped. Why had her mother?

Months later, Susan came in one day feeling depressed without knowing why. She spent the session talking about work-related issues. Near the end of the session, Susan told me that we were approaching the 50th anniversary of her mother's death, and wondered if that could be related to her vague sense of depression. Even after months of mourning, working through the layers of dissociation around her mother's suicide, the impact of this profound loss was difficult to hold onto, echoing Stern's (1983) notion of "rescuing unformulated experience from the oblivion of the familiar." Susan looked so lost at that moment, so alone, like a sad, little girl. Having survived divorce, breast cancer, depression, this motherless child stood stricken before me as she got up to leave. Spontaneously, we reached out and hugged each other and she burst into tears, letting me hold her for a few moments.

In the next session, Susan reported that she had cried for two days after our last session. She had gone for a walk that night and sat on a park bench weeping inconsolably and cried out, "I lost my mother! I lost my mother!" We talked about what it meant to Susan that I had hugged her at that moment, a spontaneous gesture perhaps evoking unconscious, somatic body memories of being held by her mother. This, in turn, unleashed both tremendous longing and heartbreaking loss. Unlike her mother, Susan had had the experience of hitting bottom and surviving, walking around in the world of intolerable pain while being held, letting go in a safe enough environment in the presence of another. Unlike her experience as a little girl (and earlier in the treatment), this time she was able to mourn her mother more freely, with an other who could now tolerate the depths of her rage and pain, so that Susan could begin to forgive her. Having gotten more deeply in touch with both love and loss, Susan poignantly reflected, "If my mother felt as bad as I did, or worse, she didn't kill herself because she didn't love me—I think she *did* love me—but she couldn't stand the pain. It was just too much to bear."

Interestingly, Susan's telling me she wanted to move to Chicago opened up the lens to the emotional abandonments that had already occurred that we had not seen clearly until now. While we had talked about her son and his struggles, we had not focused as much on aspects of their relationship that were problematic, the power struggles, the intense fighting. She was so invested in being a good mother and ashamed about her struggles with her child, that she had successfully kept this raw material out of the room, and largely out of awareness. In my unconscious identification with her, I had colluded with her in her perception that it was her toxic husband who was damaging to her son, his rage, his pathology. This was true, but not the whole story, as it also obfuscated the degree to which Susan had not sufficiently protected her son from his father's abusiveness.

On his 16th birthday, Susan gave her son a card that said, "No matter where you go, remember you'll always be loved." Her son's response was, "that's nice, but where were you all those years when dad was being abusive to me?" Susan was speechless, hurt, angry. Not wanting to be defensive or retaliatory, she said nothing. We talked about her son's sense of having been neglected, how Susan wished she could "erase" the past.

"What would you erase?" I asked.

"His hurt," she responded.

We discussed how excruciating it felt to bear witness to her son's anger and blame, to take responsibility and apologize for not being there when he had needed her protection, familiar territory for me. Perhaps Susan had been blinded to the extent of her husband's abusiveness toward herself and her son because allowing herself to experience this horror would have meant opening up access to intolerable pain in her past which she was not yet ready to face. I have enormous admiration for Susan's efforts to come to terms with the anguish she has suffered as well as the pain she has caused. In her genuine efforts to reconnect with her son, Susan has had to reckon with the tragedy of repetition while creating space for reparation and forgiveness.

The treatment continued to open up into a more flexible, affectively vibrant place as we explored themes of aliveness and deadness, presence and absence. In the transference, there was a noticeable shift from seeking approval to a search for recognition of her true self, a desire to be seen in all her complexity. With much sadness, Susan wistfully mourned the passage of time, the years she wasted in her unhappy marriage and less than fulfilling career. This led to an opening up of creativity, and a desire to take meaningful action.

Then Susan had an amazing dream: that she was on an island that was burning, a wasteland. It was terrifying. Suddenly a giant horse with wings (and brown hair!) flew down out of the sky. She climbed on its back, and they soared off over the island, finally at a safe distance from the danger, as they surveyed the horrors below ... As we analyzed the dream, Susan began to smile, then cry, and was able to articulate with intense feeling, how much her relationship to her brown-haired analyst meant to her. She talked about the relief of being able to look at her life, past and present together, with open eyes and greater perspective. She told me that what was most striking to her about the dream was that although we were soaring miles above the earth, she was not afraid. While neither Susan nor I realized it at the time, I think Susan's dream of flying poetically captures the transmutation of her unconscious identification with her mother and her mother's suicide (by jumping off a building) to a less dissociated, more painful but more authentic affective experience, flying up instead of down (Neil Altman, personal communication).

Susan decided to take a memoir writing class, and we had many conversations about how the process of writing both facilitated her access to painful memories and helped contain them, echoing Solow Glennon's (2007) notions of how the creation of "an aesthetic container is a way of channeling the chaos of pain into a potentially healing beauty and form." Interestingly, it was around this time that I began to consciously make links between my own experiences in analysis and my relationship with my son and the ways in which this resonated in my work with Susan, and I was first inspired to write this paper. Clearly there was an opening up of creativity and a capacity to play in the treatment that reverberated deeply for both of us.

A year later, Susan began taking acting classes. Acting had been a passion of hers as a child and she had shown great promise, but had been discouraged by her father from pursuing an acting career. She discovered to her delight that she was inspired by acting and received recognition from teachers, leading to an invitation to join a master class for talented actors. We discussed the importance of re-discovering acting after thirty years, realizing that she had not pursued it earlier, not only because her father had disapproved, but out of her own fear of tapping into terrifying feelings: the fear of falling apart, the fear of going crazy like her mother. She said, "I never could have articulated that years ago, but that's what it was. Acting requires me to dig deep into painful emotional territory. Therapy has freed me to go to those deeper places within myself with less fear."

This reminds me again of Danticat's notion of creating dangerously, "creating as a revolt against silence." In Susan's case, this entailed a complex process of delayed mourning, revolting against her father's and the culture's prohibitions against talking about death with children, especially back in the 1950s, and reckoning with the ways in which shame around suicide created an impenetrable wall of silence lasting into her forties. As I wrote in the introduction,

> When one cannot tell one's own story, when one's memories have forsaken them, working to reclaim one's memory and creative agency becomes a central task of psychoanalysis; making sense of one's personal, familial, and sociocultural history, becoming the storyteller of one's own life.

When I talked with Susan about my paper and asked her permission to write about our work together, I was revealing a great deal about myself, my relationship with my son, my own vulnerabilities. And yet, after 12 years of work together, we knew each other on multiple levels, both conscious and unconscious. It resonated for her that I knew something about the exquisite pain of mothering a struggling child. She told me that she had always felt my empathy for her son as well as for her, and that I had always kept him in mind in a way that mattered to her, just as my own analyst had kept *my* son in mind.

This paper was complicated to write for many reasons, including concerns about exposing my son's privacy, my patient's, my own.

I worried that Susan, a private person, wouldn't give me permission to write about our work. When I asked her, she felt moved, and more importantly, trusting of me with this delicate task in the context of a deepened therapeutic relationship. We discussed how she might *not* have felt comfortable earlier in the treatment, before the mutual opening up of creativity I described. She told me she deeply appreciated my decision to ask her permission to write about our work together, and to allow her to read the paper, reflecting on how I was being transparent in a way she never had experienced with her own parents.

When the paper was done, she wanted to read it in its entirety but felt anxious about reading it on her own, so we came up with the idea of reading the paper together in our sessions. Susan pored over it *slowly over several months*, asking questions, wanting to understand the theory as well as the clinical material. She read it twice. Sometimes the paper would evoke intense feelings or memories that she wanted to pursue, and we would follow those associations. Sometimes she would put the paper aside when she had other things on her mind. What I never *anticipated* was the degree to which Susan, whose mother committed suicide when she was four, would feel found and recognized seeing herself reflected through my eyes. Reading about *my* parental angst led both to a de-idealization of me as well as a stronger identification and intimacy. Reading the paper also evoked envy, competition, and a yearning to know me more deeply, along with frustration and sadness about the limits and boundaries of our therapeutic relationship. All this we continue to process, with many unanswered questions about the meaning and impact this will have on the treatment over time.

Not surprisingly, the paper reopened old wounds: her mother's suicide, unresolved issues with her critical father, her abandonment of her son. With her aging father, it increased her sense of what remained unspoken between them. On a recent visit, her father went on a tirade about how disappointed he was in her, how he had given her everything. Tempted to either yell at him or cry, something shifted in Susan, allowing her to shift gears with her father: "Dad, I love you." Taken aback, he responded, "Well, I love you too." "Well it doesn't always feel that way," Susan retorted. Afraid of killing him with her anger for 50 years, Susan now opened a new dialogue, disarming him with love. Reading about neglecting her son was agonizing, and yet it *resonated* for her, renewing her resolve to be there for him.

Ehrenberg (1992) describes the "intimate edge" as

> not simply at the boundary between self and other; it is also at the boundary of self-awareness .... It is a point of expanding self-discovery, at which one can become more intimate with one's own experience through the evolving relationship with the other, and then more intimate with the other as one becomes more attuned to oneself. (pp. 34–5)

My son challenged me in ways I had never been challenged before. He put me in touch with my most vulnerable selves. He, together with my analyst, gave me a gift for which I'm enormously grateful, pushing me to stretch myself beyond my limits, to open access to unbearable affects and embrace previously disowned pain. This allowed me to be more responsive to my son's pain as well as the anguish of my patients. I believe that the transformative experiences in my own analysis and subsequently, in my relationship with my son opened new possibilities in my work with Susan, helping us both free ourselves from old identifications and constraints, making possible a deeper level of vulnerability, intimacy, and mutual recognition.

References

Atlas, G. (2022). *Emotional inheritance: A therapist, her patients, and the legacy of trauma.* New York: Little, Brown Spark.

Bass, A. (2003). "E" enactments in psychoanalysis: Another medium, another message. *Psychoanalytic Dialogues*, 13: 657–675.

Benjamin, J. (2004). Beyond doer and done-to: An intersubjective view of thirdness. *Psychoanalytic Quarterly*, 73: 5–46.

Ehrenberg, D. (1992). *The Intimate Edge.* New York: Norton.

Goldberger, M. (1993). "'Bright Spot,' a Variant of "Blind Spot". *Psychoanalytic Quarterly*, 62: 270–273.

Gump, J. (2010). Reality matters: The shadow of trauma on African American subjectivity. *Psychoanalytic Psychology*, 27: 42–54.

Harris, A. (2009). You must remember this. *Psychoanalytic Dialogues*, 19: 2–21.

Jacobs, T. (1991). *The use of the self.* Madison CT: International University Press.

Kraemer, S. (1996). "Betwixt the dark and the daylight" of maternal subjectivity: Meditations on the threshold. *Psychoanalytic Dialogues*, 6: 765–791.

Kuchuck, S. (2014). *Clinical implications of the psychoanalystaslife experience: When the personal becomes professional*. London: Routledge.

Levine, L. (2016a). A mutual survival of destructiveness and its creative potential for agency and desire. *Psychoanalytic Dialogues*, 26: 36–49.

Levine, L. (2016b). Mutual vulnerability: Intimacy, violation, and the shards of trauma. *Psychoanalytic Dialogues*, 26: 571–579.

Levine, L. (2012). Into thin air: The co-construction of shame, recognition and creativity in an analytic process. *Psychoanalytic Dialogues*, 22: 456–471.

Levine, L. (2009). Transformative aspects of our own analyses and their resonance in our work with our patients. *Psychoanalytic Dialogues*, 19: 454–462.

Ogden, T. (2005). *This art of psychoanalysis*. London: Routledge.

Solow Glennon, S. (2007). Affective authenticity: Crossovers between artistic expression and the therapeutic action of psychoanalysis. Paper presented at the International Association of Relational Psychoanalysis and Psychotherapy Conference, Athens, June 2007.

Stern, D. (1983). Unformulated experience: From familiar chaos to creative disorder. Contemporary Psychoanalysis, 19: 71–99.

Stern, D., Bruschweiler-Stern, N., Harrison, A., Lyons-Ruth, K., Morgan, A, Nahum, J, Sander, L, & Tronick, E. (1998). The process of therapeutic change involving implicit knowledge: Some implications of developmental observations for adult psychotherapy. *Infant Mental Health Journal*, 19: 300–308.

Chapter 2

Into Thin Air: The Interweaving of Shame, Recognition, and Creativity in an Analytic Process

"You seem so *interested*" Julia marveled, surprised by my engagement in her creative process. She had been describing a painting she had made years ago, showing me with her hand how she had painted different parts of it, while I followed her hand with my eyes, moved by her allowing me access to her artistic process, totally "in" the process of her art-making.

An artist who is extraordinarily creative in her dreams, metaphors, and artistic vision, Julia has spent much of her life struggling to make art. From early on in treatment, I was struck by this paradox, which felt poignant and deeply compelling to me. I wondered about the barriers, the emotional risks for Julia, of making the private public, of giving expression to her richly imaginative inner life through her artwork. As the youngest child in her large, upper-middle-class White San Francisco family, she felt invisible and unheard, as if she didn't have a voice. Her parents divorced when she was quite young, and Julia felt lost in a sea of separation, remarriage, and the creation of new families. In her dynamic, intellectual family, she tended to withdraw, to opt out rather than try to compete with her siblings for their parents' and step-parents' attention. Her earliest memory is lying in her crib next to a window with the wind blowing the curtains, straining to decipher whispering voices she could not comprehend. Julia experienced her mother as mysterious and inaccessible. She did not feel mirrored or recognized by her mother, leaving Julia unsure about her own feelings or desires and how to translate those desires into action. Although Julia had loving relationships with her husband, children, and friends, self-doubts and persistent negative voices

DOI: 10.4324/9781003367475-3

undermined her ability to be as open and emotionally present as she wanted to be. She had had several initially stimulating, yet ultimately unsatisfying careers, and yearned to find professional fulfillment and pleasure in her artwork.

In the session I was describing, Julia seemed to feel momentarily recognized by me as I tracked the motion of her hand, watching her recreate the painting before my eyes. It was an intimate moment, reminiscent of early mother-infant intersubjectivity (Beebe and Lachmann, 2002; Seligman, 2009; Trevarthen, 1980), full of creative possibility. But a moment later, she became distrustful, convinced that this was just my therapeutic training and attentiveness, rather than any genuine engagement or interest on my part. It was the first of many times when I was to experience the shock of going from what felt like a moment of deep mutual resonance to feeling "dropped" by her as Julia disavowed her sense of connection with me.

This pattern of enlivening engagement followed by skepticism, disappointment, and disengagement was repeated over several years, and Julia and I tried to deconstruct it from multiple perspectives. We went through periods in the treatment in which there was a shared sense of vivacity, a creative sense of "flow" in sessions, in which she imagined and described art projects she wanted to create. We would both feel hopeful and optimistic about her capacity to make art. But inevitably, the aliveness would disappear, as if into thin air, and she would shift into a more discouraged state, in which her art felt far away and inaccessible. At such times, she would periodically consider stopping treatment.

The sense that the aliveness disappeared "as if into thin air" was quite disappointing and unsettling to both of us, and there was something uncanny about how it surprised us *each time it happened*. Over time, I became aware of how this moment of mutual dysregulation led to a whole sequence of intrapsychic responses on my part; in particular, a sense of loss on multiple levels. I felt disappointed for Julia each time, sensing that she had been *on the verge* of getting to a more sustained, creative place. I held the hope of her getting to that place even when she couldn't, even when she felt hopeless and despairing. And yet, it still felt like a palpable loss to me. I missed the shared, mutual pleasure of vitality and creativity, and I was aware of feeling grateful to Julia for the opportunity to feel like my most creative self as an analyst, with greater access to my own imagination and affective states as they related to her experience. Could I hold onto my *own* liveliness and creativity in the absence of hers? Each time she considered ending therapy, Julia subtly or more directly devalued the treatment and the importance of our connection, and I was aware of feeling "dropped" in the face of the threat of the loss of our relationship. And yet, I fought for it. I believed in Julia, in the value of our work together—and in the possibility of her attaining a more sustained inspiration and creativity.

As I became aware of this pattern, I wondered with Julia about what triggered these shifts between vitality and flatness, creativity and despair, and talked with her about the importance of understanding the dynamics underlying it. Over time, we began to see a connection between the dyadic engagement/disengagement and an opening or closing down of aliveness and access to her own creative process. We also came to understand the shifts from imagination and creativity to discouragement and hopelessness as intersubjective and co-created. Julia felt a deep longing for recognition, yet when she experienced that connection with me, it felt unfamiliar, difficult to trust.

There was a sense of feeling momentarily held and then dropped, leading to a sense of shame and a "crashing" of self, and despair. Immediately following those moments of connection, perhaps unconsciously I became her preoccupied, unavailable mother who could not be relied upon for affective recognition, and she reacted, understandably, with mistrust and anger. I too felt a sense of shame for experiencing and trusting in the mutual connection and then having it denied by her. It felt as if she was pulling the rug out from under me, or perhaps, out from under both of us! This too would be repeated over time in the treatment, before we could understand and deconstruct it in a meaningful way, and before we could recognize and name the critical role of shame in the dynamic.

In this chapter, I will raise questions about both intrapsychic and intersubjective dynamics that open or close down vitality and creativity in our work with patients. I will explore ways in which patients' access to their imagination, dreams, and other unconscious realms may be intimately connected to the analyst's variable and shifting receptivity to her own imagination and creativity and consider the ways in which creativity is both solitary and co-constructed. Furthermore, I will consider the powerful impact of shame on the creative process, both intrapsychically, blocking access to memory, and leading to the negative, critical voices that block one's capacity to create art; and intersubjectively, how "shame can travel insidiously across relational realms, passed back and forth, alternately projected and introjected, from analyst to patient" and back again, deadening spontaneity, imagination, and creativity. I will illustrate how shame is such a toxic experience, it undoes us. And yet, there is also the possibility for detoxifying shame thru the analytic process that has the potential for creative growth.

Shame and Recognition

Alan Schore (2003) refers to shame as "the primary social emotion," emerging at around 14–16 months in the context of the parent-infant relationship. He describes how the toddler, with excitement and elation, looks to the caregiver to share and mirror her joy, and if this attunement does not occur, the toddler experiences a sense of shame: "The ensuing break in an anticipated visual-affective communication triggers a shock-induced deflation of positive affect … and shame represents this rapid state transition from a pre-existing positive state to a negative state" (p. 17). Shore elaborates further that this is emotionally dys-regulating for the child and experienced as a discontinuity in the child's "going on being" (Winnicott, 1958). What follows is that "elation, heightened arousal, and elevated activity level instantly evaporate … and (the toddler) becomes inhibited and strives to avoid attention in order to become 'unseen'" (p.18).

Reading Shore's description of the elated toddler who looks eagerly to the parent to share in her delight, but is met instead with a lack of empathy or mirroring, one can imagine how Julia learned to be invisible and unheard, an adaptive defense against shame. One can also hear echoes, antecedents of the pattern that emerged between us in the treatment, the shifts between aliveness and deadness, creativity and despair, the shock, and dys-regulation that followed the loss and disavowal of mutuality and connection.

Bromberg (1998) describes the crucial role of enactments in working analytically with shame, asserting that:

> for individuals experiencing intense shame, no words can capture the assaultive intensity of the experience. It is only through

reliving the trauma through enactment with the analyst that its magnitude can be known by an "other," hopefully this time an "other" who will have the courage to participate in the reliving while simultaneously holding the patient's psychological safety as a matter of prime concern. (p. 296)

However, there's psychological risk for analyst as well as patient as the "re-living" is enacted *between* them. The analyst must learn about the patient's experiences with shame from the inside out, embodying the role of victim as well as perpetrator (Davies, 1999, 2004). In the moment when I feel dropped by Julia, I am the in-attentive mother, and seconds later, the shamed child.

Winnicott believed that being *seen* by the mother is being "recognized for who one is" and that "not to be seen by the mother, at least at the moment of the spontaneous gesture, is not to exist" (Phillips, 1988, p. 130). Winnicott (1967) described how the mother's responsiveness to the infant's bids for attention and recognition lead to the development of her sense of self. When the mother or caregiver resonates and responds to the infant's spontaneous gesture, what had been a random movement becomes endowed with meaning, a communication, a basic aspect of empathy and intersubjectivity. Winnicott (1967) also believed that the capacity for play and creativity develops within the context of the mother-infant relationship, and is related to seeing and being seen. He stated that "being seen is at the basis of creative looking" (p. 114) and that when babies look into their mothers' faces and do not see themselves reflected back "their own creative capacity begins to atrophy" (p. 112).

In an intriguing paper, "Temporality and spontaneity in infancy and psychoanalysis," Seligman (2009) captures this intricate dance of mother-infant interaction, describing how a mother's attuned response to her infant's spontaneous gesture "essentially transforms the movement over time and space" to create intersubjective communication and meaning. This gives the baby "compelling evidence of her effect on the world." This sense of intentionality, of having an impact was something that Julia was searching for, as she grew up feeling invisible, "like a ghost." She had a strong desire to "embody" herself more, to feel more enlivened and connected to her own feelings as well as closer to others. I will come back to this issue later in the chapter when I discuss what it meant to Julia to see that she could have a deep, emotional effect on me. According to Seligman, when a mother is not responsive to an infant's gestures, "there is no sense of time moving forward," only "the stasis of a present which never gives way to an emergent future." (p. 5–8)

In exploring the intersubjective nature of mutual recognition, there is also the question of the parent's subjectivity (Benjamin, 1990) and the power of mirroring the spontaneous gesture for the parent as well as the child. In the novel, *What I Loved*, by Siri Hustvedt, an 11-year-old child dies, and the father, deep in mourning, immerses himself in the artwork of his creative and talented son. The father, an art historian, begins to trace the lines of his son's drawings, and finds it enormously evocative, both comforting and heartbreaking. The father reflects, "I found the motion of his living hand that way, and once I had started it, I couldn't stop" (p. 146).

This vignette brings to mind recent research on mirror neurons (Gallese, 2004, 2009) which suggests that we have empathic resonance to others at a deep, bodily level. It reflects the ways in which action itself becomes a way of knowing the other, experiencing the other on a visceral, embodied level. Gallese (2004) writes:

> The shared intersubjective space in which we live from birth continues long afterward to constitute a substantial part of our semantic space. When we observe other acting individuals, facing their full range of *expressive* power (the way they act, the emotions and feelings they display), a meaningful embodied inter-individual link is automatically established … . Sensations and emotions displayed by others can also be empathized with, and therefore implicitly understood, through a neural matching mechanism. (p. 15)

Building on Winnicott's and Bion's notions of play and dreaming, Ogden (2009) suggests that

> when an analysis is a "going concern" (Winnicott, 1964), the patient and analyst are able to engage, both individually and with one another, in a process of dreaming. The area of "overlap" of the patient's dreaming and the analyst's dreaming is the place where analysis occurs (Winnicott, 1971, p. 38).
>
> (Ogden, 2009, p. 14)

In his book, *Rediscovering psychoanalysis: Thinking and Dreaming, Learning and Forgetting*, Ogden is evoking a broader, poetic notion of "dreaming," referring to a state of being, and a way of listening, that's open and receptive to the unconscious of both patient and analyst. The essence of this analytic process is to help the patient become more fully alive to his experience, or as Ogden felicitously suggests, "dreaming himself more fully into existence" (p. 17).

Julia and Me

Throughout my work with Julia, her dreams have been a rich source of creativity and inspiration, giving us access to multiple layers of memory and desire. Early on, Julia had a dream that has evolved into a central metaphor in our work. In the dream, she is sitting outside a house on a porch. There are wild, lush, beautiful plants growing underneath the porch, peeking through the slats, but unable to grow or develop, to see the light of day. One of Julia's primary reasons for seeking therapy was to feel more in touch with her affective, unconscious, and creative selves. Through this dream, we wonder about how she protected herself as a child by cutting off her feelings, shielding herself from pain. We wonder too about the lush plants growing underneath the porch as her creative spontaneous gestures, which were never recognized, appreciated, or nurtured, never given a chance to grow and develop.

Through this dream, Julia and I also begin to consider her creative blocks as a *lack of access* to the creativity within her as opposed to an *absence* of creativity, which feels like a relief and a revelation, though difficult to hold onto. The ongoing challenge then becomes opening access to her rich and lively imagination and fantasy life, and drawing from that reservoir in order to create art. We talk about reframing blocks to artistic creation as caused by anxiety rather than a lack of ideas, and discover, in the process, that the notion of "access" is a potentially powerful vehicle to tuning into, trusting and valuing one's creative voice.

Frequently artists and writers get stuck in the act of creating out of a fear of lack of originality, the sense that everything they want to create has been said or done before. I believe we each possess a unique and highly personal voice, so that our expression or rendering of a particular piece of art has the potential to offer a fresh perspective if one is open to one's own authentic experience and courageous enough to allow one's "little voices" to have a life of their own. Over the years, Julia and I have come back again and again to this metaphor of the lush growth under the porch. We've wondered how to understand and deconstruct this porch that not only provides a respite from the chaos inside the house but also blocks access to her creative source and renders her invisible and outside the flow of her family.

Months later, Julia has two more dreams that reflect a blockage or difficulty gaining access to her own creativity, yet they also reveal an increased comfort with intimacy. In the first dream, Julia is with her step-father at a fancy dinner party in his house, the kind of family party where she always felt uncomfortable and invisible. Yet she's aware of feeling an unusual ease talking with him. They go outside together, and begin to dig up a huge football field where they find remarkable ancient artwork deep underground, including a huge sculpture with hieroglyphics. In the dream, Julia experiences a new sense of intimacy with her step-father. This increased comfort with herself and with him leads to a creative, underground journey and access to an inner imaginative source. Julia associates to the huge underground sculpture with hieroglyphics, the necessity of digging deep together to find her creative source, the inscrutability of the hieroglyphics, of understanding her blocks to making art. We talk about the transferential aspects of the dream, the relationship between our increasing intimacy and her access to her internal world. In another dream, there's a palpable desire for closeness and friendship with me, but a blocking of access here too. Julia and I are hanging out together in her kitchen talking; it feels good and close, until an older woman comes downstairs and shames her (perhaps both of us?) for the desire for a deeper connection. We wonder about issues of loyalty and competition, the various risks of our deepening intimacy. We talk about how this dream feels significant as a conscious desire for closeness *with me,* which can now be talked about for the first time, but it's still tinged with shame and followed by doubt, similar to the clinical vignette at the beginning of the paper.

Julia and I also discuss the importance of valuing, honoring the *experience* of vitality and imagination in its own right, the intrinsic rewards of creativity. We talk about the possibility of appreciating her imagination and artistic capacity without judgment or criticism; not evaluating the art object per se, but opening access to her own creative source. Mikaly Csikszentmihalyi (1990) writes about the concept of "flow," which he defines as an effortless, yet highly focused consciousness in which one becomes so involved in an activity that it feels spontaneous, a process of discovery. Csikszentmihalyi and his colleagues interviewed artists and poets, rock climbers and skiers, scientists and philosophers across diverse cultures; all describing this sense of "flow" in a similar way, becoming one with the action one is performing, which is intrinsically rewarding, an end in itself. There is a lack of self-consciousness or fear of failure and a distorted sense of time, as one gets lost in the moment, fully present and alive.

Jackson Pollock, the Abstract Expressionist painter, articulates this sense of "flow" in describing the process of his art-making:

> When I am *in* my painting, I'm not aware of what I'm doing. It is only after a sort-of "get acquainted" period that I see what I have been about. I have no fears about making changes, destroying the image, etc, because the painting has a life of its own. I try to let it come through.
>
> (Anfam, 1990, p. 125)

This notion of flow embodied by Pollock is also central to Ghent's (1990) conception of surrender, a striving toward self-expansion and creativity, "an experience of being 'in the moment,' totally in the present, where past and future, the two tenses that require 'mind' in the sense of secondary processes, have receded from consciousness" (p. 111).

When I mention the notion of "flow" to Julia, she has read about it, knows exactly what I am referring to. When I ask her if she has ever experienced that state of "flow," she replies, "Last weekend, when I was making pig soup." She describes how she became immersed in the act of making soup, trusting herself completely, as she added various ingredients: no onions, garlic, lots of pepper, without questioning herself, without all the negative voices interfering with the process of creating this delicious soup. Julia tells me that she experiences cooking, feeding her family and friends, as inventive and generative. It doesn't have all the emotional baggage that art has for her. The myriad critical voices in her head are silent when she cooks.

This brings to mind Marion Milner's (1957) book, *On Not Being Able to Paint*, in which Milner explores the mysteries and complexity of artistic freedom and impasse. Through her self-analysis and "free drawings," Milner bridges the worlds of psychoanalysis and art, seeking to understand the artistic process and free herself of creative inhibitions. In the conclusion, Milner makes a striking statement:

> Observations of problems to do with painting had all led up to the idea that awareness of the external world is itself a creative process, an immensely complex creative exchange between what comes from inside and what comes from outside. (p. 146)

Writing in the 1950s, Milner did not have a language or relational framework in which to understand the radical implications of her experiential, creative journey for an intersubjective model of creativity and psychoanalysis open to the interpenetrating subjectivities of patient and analyst.

At times, Julia begins an art project, only to abandon it early on when she feels dissatisfied with it in some way. We discuss the importance of making use of ruthlessness and destruction in the act of creating (Winnicott, 1969), the willingness to throw away work that is not authentic or true, and the difficulty of not being too attached to ideas that don't flow, as they can stand in the way of taking creative leaps forward. We talk about the enormous difficulty of being ruthless with one's work without being ruthless toward oneself. For Julia, the fear of making art that is "no good" stops her in her tracks, keeps her from even getting started. And when she does allow herself to create art, the challenge is finding a way to hold onto what's good and true while discarding the bad.

But even with all this exploration, playfulness, dreaming, analyzing her defenses around making art, imagining art projects, and sharing ideas with me, Julia still wasn't making art, or seeing it through to completion. Even though we seemed to be gaining insight into the dynamics underlying the shifts from aliveness and creativity to deadness and discouragement, she continued to get stuck in the *act* of making art. She struggled to authorize herself as an artist. And that was discouraging to her and continued to bring her down, triggering the more hopeless, depressed states in sessions.

Around this time, however, a couple of years into therapy, Julia got involved professionally in a new creative project which has taken off and grown in exciting directions under her leadership. While this was exhilarating and, and at times, deeply satisfying to her, she was bothered by the fact that the project was not her original conception, her baby, and still yearned to make art of her own, to create something from the ground up. In addition to the creative aspects of the work itself, Julia also enjoyed the communal aspects of the project, working with imaginative, resourceful colleagues who engaged and inspired each other.

As she was feeling closer to me and beginning to gain more confidence in her creative self, Julia decided to show me some of her drawings. I felt quite moved that she wanted to show me her artwork after all the time we've spent talking about her struggles in this area. She seemed genuinely engaged too, taking pleasure in my responses and appreciation of her work. I looked forward to processing this intimate, shared experience in our next meeting.

But in the following session, Julia had a completely different perception and memory of our interaction. She was angry with me, devaluing of my artistic aesthetic, once again distrustful of my interest and appreciation of her art. She disavowed the mutual connection I had felt so palpably, asserting that I had only told her what I believed she wanted and needed to hear, just doing my therapeutic duty. I felt shocked, abandoned, confused, and affectively destabilized by having an experience seemingly shared with her, so flatly denied by her. It was an even more amplified example of what Shore describes as feeling unrecognized and dropped, an experience leading to shame. In fact, I felt unrecognized on two profound levels: both in my own affective perceptions and in the mutual and disavowed connection with her. Although we struggled to process and deconstruct this enactment over several weeks, it still felt like something was missing, unsettled, like we were not getting to the heart of the matter.

In retrospect, I think that there was something important in how we both held our ground, maintaining our different versions of what had happened, as we tried to build a tenuous bridge between us. While I did not submit to her disavowal of the intimacy and mutual connection, I tried to stay open and curious about her response to sharing her artwork with me. I wondered aloud about the ways in which she may have felt exposed or intruded upon by my appreciative responses to her artwork. Most importantly, I survived her aggression and devaluation of me and our work together (Ghent, 1992; Winnicott, 1969). But, all the while, I struggled to process my own feelings of abandonment and disappointment; feeling once again, unrecognized and dropped by Julia.

Even though I did not yet understand why we continued to re-enact this dynamic, I knew intuitively that it was meaningful and needed to be deconstructed, creating potential space for each of our subjectivities. I also surmised that Julia was communicating something critical through this enactment about her own unmetabolized, painful relational experience that she needed me to understand experientially, that hadn't yet been verbalized (Bass, 2003, 2009). Aron (2003) suggests that "enactments may well be a central means by which patients and analysts enter into each other's inner world and discover themselves as participants within each other's psychic life, mutually constructing the relational matrix that constitutes the medium of psychoanalysis" (p. 629).

And then I realized in retrospect, years after many years of supervision with Philip Bromberg, that in being empathic toward one part of Julia, the part that wanted/needed affirmation of her creative self, I was unrecognizing or abandoning of another. I was too appreciative and excited about her artistic self, and her desire to share it with me. I was not in touch with the part of her that had sought therapy for her lifelong struggle to find her creative voice, who felt unseen and unheard, the lonely baby in the crib, straining to decipher whispering voices she could not comprehend.

Bromberg writes:

There are times ... when the therapist thinks he has had a good hour and the patient leaves and comes back feeling awful, and the therapist doesn't know what happened. From my perspective, one part of the patient's self has felt unacknowledged. The part that is committed to preservation and the protection of the dissociative structure is feeling unappreciated, alienated, and endangered by all this new "wonderful" change that's going on. It feels to that part of the patient's self as if the therapist doesn't want it around, so you hear a voice from this dissociated self-state reminding the therapist not to get too carried away by his own therapeutic skill. It is in effect saying, "You think that everything is OK because you had a good session, but *I* am not OK; *I* am very scared."

(Bromberg, 2000, pp. 24–25)

This quote wonderfully captures what I believe happened with Julia and me in this session when she shared her artwork with me.

In a session soon afterward, when she has been talking about trying to engage her father in a conversation about her life and creative work, and he was disinterested and critical, Julia identifies her emotional response as one of shame. Julia tells me that she made herself vulnerable by sharing a creative part of herself, only to have this spontaneous gesture go unrecognized by her father—yet again—and how that triggered a sense of shame in her. As I listen closely, I gradually become aware that shame is exactly what I had felt with *her*, when she disavowed the powerful, intersubjective connection between us, both in the session when she created the painting before my eyes and in the session after she showed me her drawings. Should I share this awareness of my own countertransference with her? Will it open potential space or feel intrusive, too much of my own sub-jectivity, derail the treatment? This feels akin to what Stern et al. (1998) describe as a "now moment," a unique moment of opportunity where analyst and patient "are meeting as persons relatively un-hidden by their usual therapeutic roles" and their actions "cannot be routine, habitual, or technical" (p. 912).

I take a risk; decide to share my feelings with her. I tell her that as she was describing feeling unrecognized and shamed by her father, I realized that shame is exactly what *I had felt* when she disavowed the shared intimacy and connection between us as she showed me her drawings. Julia is taken aback, and begins to cry, so rare for her. At first, she feels concerned about hurting me, about evoking in me, an affect that is deeply familiar to her over a lifetime, the shame that she dreads. Then, as we explore her responses, she speaks of feeling grateful that I would share my own vulnerability with her, moved that she could have such an impact on me, and that I trusted her enough to tell her. For Julia, who had grown up feeling invisible and unheard, feeling like she could have an impact on me, that I could survive her aggression and not retaliate, and even more than that, be *changed* by her, was a revelation.

This session felt transformative for both of us, a pivotal point in the treatment. There was something about my taking an emotional risk, *a leap of faith perhaps*, by being open and vulnerable with Julia about her impact on me that allowed Julia to let her guard down as well (Ehrenberg, 1992, 1996).

Julia had taken a risk with her father too, by talking with him from a more authentic, creative self, and had been shamed in the process by his lack of attunement. It was not, however, until the moment when she identified her response to her father as one of shame, that I became aware of my own shame in response to her disavowal of our mutual connection. Her defensive identification with her father, which led to her shaming me clearly constituted an enactment in the form of a projective identification.

I am taking a relational view of projective identification as an unconscious, powerful *communication* of a split-off, intolerable affective experience that needs to be experienced by another, so that it can be put into words and worked through (Aron, 2003; Benjamin, 2004, 2009, 2010; Bromberg, 2006; Cooper, 2000, 2004; Davies, 2004; Ehrenberg, 1992, 1996; Hoffman, 1998). This is a further elaboration of the Kleinian conception of disavowed, dreaded affects evacuated by the patient into the analyst that need to be contained and metabolized privately by the analyst. However, although there was a shift within post-Kleinian theory from projective identification as a *defense* to projective identification as a *communication* (Rosenfeld, 1987), it is still currently a given within the Kleinian tradition that the analyst never discloses her subjective experience of the projective identification, as this would constitute "an act of merger and fails to honor the separateness of patient and analyst (Cooper, 2004, p. 544). Relational and interpersonal analysts have expanded the notion of projective identification, which Mitchell (1993) refers to as "the interpersonalization of projective identification" (p. 79).

By making the clinical choice to share my countertransference with Julia, I was building on a relational model of projective identification in which analysts may choose to disclose aspects of their subjective experience in order to create potential space to reflect on the co-creation of an enactment with the patient. As Benjamin (2010) suggested,

> By expanding her sense of the frame, the analyst can recover from dysregulation well enough to contain and use enactment. The degree to which this is possible ... depends on the gradual creation of the intersubjective space for reflection, mutual regulation, recognition of vulnerability and humor. Thus contained, enactment can afford analysts an opportunity to engage in joint reflection with patients, to share the revelation of process in thinking about them or feeling with them. In addition, it may afford the patient an opportunity to be effective, so that not only the patient but also the analyst changes. (Slavin and Kriegman, 1998, p. 116–117)

I believe that Julia was communicating something critical through this enactment about her own unmetabolized, painful, relational experience that she needed me to understand *from the inside out* (Bass, 2003, 2009; Levine, 2009a,b). However, it took many repetitions of this enactment between us, some quite subtle, others more charged, before Julia could get through to me, before I could begin to understand this dynamic as a projective identification. As Bromberg (2006) suggested, dissociated, "not-me" self-states continue to get enacted in the treatment until they are experienced in the countertransference and gradually understood by analyst and patient.

Stern et al. (1998) suggest that the "open space" following a "now moment" between mothers and infants or analysts and patients holds the potential for creativity. Now moments "leave in their wake an 'open space' in which a shift in the intersubjective environment creates a new equilibrium ... Creativity becomes possible as the patient's 'implicit relational knowing' has been freed of constraints imposed by the habitual" (p. 914). For Julia, recognizing that she can have an emotional impact on me seems to shift something significant in the treatment, creating intersubjective space, and opening the possibility for a deeper intimacy between us (Ehrenberg, 1992, 1996; Seligman, 2009).

In his discussion of this paper in *Psychoanalytic Dialogues*, Philip Ringstrom (2012) adds another layer to understanding this enactment around shame from an intersubjective perspective, building on Benjamin's idea of the moral third. He writes:

> [Levine] systematically spreads the impact of shame over the shoulders of the dyad, without locating it in one or the other (Ringstrom, 2012) … It is precisely this mode of engagement that restores the dyad's capacity to play with their ideas, … adhering to Benjamin's (2004) idea of the "moral third" in which the analyst both takes responsibility for the impact of her subjectivity on the patient's and enables the patient to grasp her impact on the analyst. In this manner, … shame moves from being the enemy of creativity to an informant of how it truncates that process in both, without either one ending up "holding the bag."

Julia and I now begin to explore more deeply the powerful impact of shame on her memory and sense of self, how the lack of mirroring and recognition she received led her to disavow psychic pain and minimize her impact on others, as well as blocking access to her creative potential. Julia came into therapy convinced that she had a terrible memory, and concerned that, as she aged, she was losing whatever memory she did have, like her mother, who is in her nineties. For a long time, Julia had trouble accessing childhood memories, particularly of one-on-one time with her mother. The recollections she did have were mostly alone or with her siblings, or with her parents present, but emotionally inaccessible.

But, as we begin to access and deconstruct the degree of shame that she internalized at any early age, more specific memories of her mother and their time together become available to her. Julia and I begin to weave together a shared narrative history about her early life, especially with her mother: her mother's cool detachment, her unpredictable anger, Julia's anxious sense of never knowing which mother she would find. Julia remembers her efforts to get her mother's attention; performing for her and her friends at cocktail hour, waking up from scary dreams and sleeping curled up outside her parent's bedroom door, yearning to be comforted, but afraid of her mother's anger at being awakened in the middle of the night.

As Julia is able to gain access to memories, her perceptions of her mother are changing as well. Other narratives are emerging. Julia visits her mom, who, suffering from Alzheimer's, literally does not recognize her. But to Julia's surprise, there is a peacefulness as they listen to Ella Fitzgerald together, while her mother lies in bed. Julia tells me, it's almost like they are mother and baby, but with the roles reversed. These benign, quiet moments of joining, the experience of being alone in the presence of another (Winnicott, 1958) are reminiscent of her most intimate childhood memory with her mother: reading silently together, each with her own book, in their living room, not talking or interacting, just being together.

Coming to terms with the "lack" in parenting and the pain it caused is allowing Julia to mourn the mother she didn't have, the idealized mother. She is beginning to forgive her mother and make peace with her limitations, to recognize what *is* possible to share in their remaining time together (Harris, 2009; Loewald, 1979). As Harris (2009) suggests, "Return and repetition are always elements of change ... There is melancholy, a sense of loss and sadness that weaves through change" (Harris, 2009, p. 4).

Soon afterward, Julia is again feeling discouraged about her difficulties creating art, even though she has a clear vision of two new sculptures she wants to make, and has begun them both before getting stuck once again. We reflect on her dream about the underground sculpture with hieroglyphics, talk about familiar issues of obstacles to making art, critical voices in her head, the fear of throwing herself into the act of creating and discovering she can't do it, feeling like a fraud. We discuss the risks of allowing herself to become enlivened in a sustained way, open to her own creativity and desires; the risks of being intimate with others, with me. How allowing herself to experience hope and desire is inherently risky (Mitchell, 1993), filled with the possibility, the inevitability of loss (Harris, 2009).

Julia then speaks of shame, and its connection to not being "recognized" as a child, which we've been exploring. Sadly, she begins to talk about not feeling recognized by any of the adults in her family, and recalls her earliest memory of being in a crib all alone, hearing the whispering unintelligible voices from the wind blowing the curtains. I feel immersed in her sadness, resonate with her grief. Then, there is a noticeable shift in her self-state as Julia, deflated and dispirited, questions the accuracy of her memory, the reality of her childhood pain. *How bad was it really*? Having been down this road together many times before, this time it feels like familiar territory and I pick up on her shift in self-states, and ask her about it. This childhood narrative where Julia allows herself to experience and acknowledge to me the depths of her pain and loneliness is new and fragile, vulnerable to being closed down and disavowed by the shame it evokes in the recalling and re-telling. As we deconstruct what happened between us, we can both see how my resonating with her pain led her to doubt her own experience, to distrust the accuracy of her memory.

It is almost the end of the session and Julia mentions to me that she has spoken to her teenage daughter who is struggling with anxiety. Julia had asked me for a referral for her several months ago and the therapy seemed to be going well. Julia tells me that her daughter is considering increasing her sessions from once to twice a week.

Julia says, "I told her to let herself go where she needs to go, and just be *in* the experience, to get the help she needs."

"You were so recognizing of her experience," I reply. "You're giving her what you didn't get as a kid."

Julia (tentatively):　　"Yeah, I guess I was ... I'm not always so attuned though ... I guess it feels good to do that for her now. I can see that it's helping." As she got ready to leave, she added, "And you're helping me."

In the next session, Julia tells me that she's still feeling down, discouraged. She looks sadder than I've ever seen her, and I comment on her sadness. She begins to cry. After a few moments, she says that she thinks she's sad about her mother, who really never got what she wanted—to feel a connection with other people—and now she has lost her chance. This is a striking moment to me, since when I've asked Julia in the past about her feelings about her mother's loss of memory, and her literal inability to recognize Julia in the past few years, Julia has expressed some sadness about her mother's deterioration, but it has felt distant and muted. Generally, she has been matter-of-fact, glad to be able to care for her mother in whatever ways she can. Now, in her sadness, Julia acknowledges that she's afraid of becoming her mother, and then relates an amazing dream from the night before:

> *Julia finds a little, round plant on the ground and breaks it open, and inside she finds what appears to be a burr, but turns out to be a baby owl. She picks up the owl and it begins to grow as she holds it close against her body, until it's the size of a human baby. Then she finds herself at the Stone Club, an exclusive country club that her family belonged to as a child. Still holding the owl, she's approached by a WASPY blond woman who offers her a job there, which she declines. She has no interest in being part of this club, this world. Then the woman walks up to a little girl who looks very sad and neglected. The woman surprises Julia by being warm and nurturing to the little girl.*

Julia says she thinks that both the WASPY woman and the little girl are parts of herself. The fact that she so clearly identifies with the sad, lonely little girl feels like a milestone, an embracing of her childhood pain that she has disavowed for so long. She worries about whether she's cold like her mother, yet the woman surprises her with her empathy and tenderness. The woman also offers her a job, which Julia declines, having "no interest" in being part of this club that is "made of stone." We wonder about the woman surprising Julia with her warmth as reflective of Julia's evolving perspective on her mother, opening up memories of what her mother could and did give to her emotionally as well as what was missing. This dream seems to hold worlds of meaning that I imagine we will continue to process for a long time.

There is a mutuality in the nurturing of the owl, a maternal protectiveness that fills Julia with love and warmth, a feeling that stays with her all day after she awakens from the dream. She tells me that the baby owl might represent both her children whom she has loved and nurtured as well as her art, for which she continues to try to create transitional space. We play with notions of who I am in the dream—the cold woman who can surprise her with my empathy and affection? The mother who embraces the baby owl who grows from cold (burr/brrr) to warm as she's held? But, can I be trusted? Or, perhaps, the mutuality in the nurturing of the owl represents the vitality and creativity we experience together when the treatment feels alive and inspired, or the (owl-like) wisdom that grows out of our shared exploration. And what about the sad, neglected little girl?

Then, Julia associates to an old dream, which we have talked about before, about a three-year-old girl lying dead in a pond. But this time, for the first time, Julia begins to cry with real anguish. She feels despairing, and I resonate, deeply, with her pain. I experience her sense of *drowning* in the sadness, how agonizing it feels to be in this emotional place. Then, we are quiet together. I tell her that it's taken us so long to get to this old and deep pain, to allow herself to own it and not discount it, that it feels important to honor it, make space for it. She doesn't disagree. We talk about how there had been no room for her pain growing up, no recognition of her loneliness, her sense of invisibility.

Julia shares with me that she is aware of "a split reaction." "Part of me knows that what you're saying feels true and right," she says. "Another part is saying, 'Oh, that's just therapy-speak—don't listen to that.'" It feels significant that at this point, Julia can tell this to me, can reflect on these two self-states, one old, one new and vulnerable. Instead of being only in the cynical, distrusting self-state and responding from that place, which would have re-enacted our old familiar dance, she is beginning to "stand in the spaces," as Bromberg (1998) describes, to build bridges between self-states. A moment later, Julia looks me in the eye, and tells me she is starting to trust me, to believe what I'm saying, to take in my faith in her. A powerful, shared moment. As she is getting up to leave, Julia finds a small, blank, white sticker on her lap. "A price tag ... but it has no price on it," she notes with curiosity. (PAUSE) "Priceless," she says with a smile. She walks over to me, gently sticks it on my forehead, and walks out the door.

I am enormously touched by this gesture, which feels simultaneously intimate, playful, and mischievous. Julia takes a risk by spontaneously reaching out, physically and emotionally, irreverently crossing boundaries, trusting that I will receive this gift in the generous spirit in which it was offered.

Thinking about my session with Julia later, I reflect on how the edge of growth is always vulnerable. I have an association to a conversation with a friend who is an artist (G. Fearey, personal communication) about meristems, the tip of a plant that is the most tender and vulnerable, yet has the fastest growing cells, and leads to new growth, which is necessary for the plant's survival. If you remove or damage the meristem, you truncate the plant's growth. This feels connected to many conversations Julia and I have had about the complexity of going to deep, painful places, which triggers shame and anguish, yet simultaneously recognizing that this is also the source of her creative process.

As Julia walks into a recent session, I notice a lightness and ease in the way she carries herself, a playfulness and warmth in her eyes. She is delighted about a recent article in the *New York Times* in which she has been interviewed about the artistic project that she has led and nurtured at work. The project has continued to grow in innovative ways, and she now feels a stronger sense of ownership and pride in this endeavor. The article feels like a momentous affirmation of her achievement and hard work in a creative realm. We talk about how she is beginning to develop a new relationship to creative obstacles. In the past, obstacles derailed her, stopping her in her tracks. Recently, she has begun to see them as problems to be solved, rather than mountains that cannot be moved.

When I ask Julia's permission to write about our work together, tell her that I am writing a paper about creativity, she is thrilled. She says, in reflecting on our work together, "I had the thought that a river runs through it." Julia is quiet for a few moments. Then, I have an association that I share with her about a recent New York Times article about kayaking and the removal of hundreds of dams built in the 1950s and 1960s because they are getting too old, outliving their usefulness. The kayakers are thrilled about new whitewater adventures, and the excitement of uncharted territory, not knowing what the removal of the dams will bring.

When I tell Julia that I have finished writing the paper, she asks if she can read it. We talk about what she imagines it will feel like to read my creative work, particularly a paper describing our psychoanalytic journey, when she has struggled so much with authorizing herself as an artist. Would she feel used or intruded upon even though she had given me permission to write about our therapy? What I sense from Julia is more curiosity and excitement, as well as some anxiety about how I will depict her and our work together. She also describes feeling a joint sense of ownership of our therapy, that in some way extends to the creation of my paper.

I email Julia the paper with an uneasy mix of anticipation and trepidation. As the next session approaches, my anxiety rises. I hope she will feel seen and recognized in my description of our work together, but I dread a repetition of our old dynamic of shame, anger, and devaluation, notwithstanding all the work we have done around this issue. I wonder whether I will once again be dropped by her. Selfishly, I worry that Julia might rescind her permission for me to write the paper, while knowing that my first obligation is to her and the analysis.

To my great relief, Julia enters the next session, holding my paper (like the owl) against her chest, and looks me straight in the eye. "It's amazing," she says. "I had no idea how personal it was going to be. It's a story—my story—and you and I are the main characters. It's authentic and honest, and you were so open about your own vulnerability. That surprised me." She pauses, shyly.

> I didn't realize how much you cared about me … I know, that's exactly what the paper is about, about how I wasn't recognized as a child, that it's been so hard for me to accept it when I am recognized. Like when I would see a sympathetic look in your eye when I was talking about something painful, I would immediately distrust it, distrust *you*. And doubt my own experience and memory.

Julia then tells me that when she began to read the paper on her computer, she went through it and changed all the "Julia's" to her real name, to see herself reflected in the narrative. "Reading it was so powerful," she continues. "It's a beautiful story, not idealized, but not critical either—not that I thought it would be." She laughs. "It's such an authentic recognition of me, and of our work together, … a gift."

Julia tells me she has begun taking pottery classes, and that after a great first class, she had two disappointing classes in which the clay kept falling off the wheel. Rather than getting discouraged and giving up, Julia practiced in the studio for two hours before her next class. She describes listening to the experienced potters discussing technique, aware of feeling surprisingly comfortable and un-self-conscious, instead of intimidated and self-critical. Julia then shows me with her hands how her teacher covered Julia's hands with her own so she could feel the correct way to sculpt the clay on the wheel. She tells me she loved the visceral feeling of her hands on the clay, the teacher's hands on hers; and that this embodied experience stayed with her all day.

Julia says, "The barrier between me and other people is dissolving." I feel this. We reflect on how much more comfortable she feels asking for and receiving help, allowing herself to touch and be touched. This is leading to a more sustained, less ephemeral sense of emotional freedom, spontaneity, and engagement in her relationships with family and friends, as well as greater access to herself and her creative voice. She is still working on authorizing herself as an artist, but she seems more sanguine about making art of her own, as her work has become a vehicle to express her creative vision. It seems only fitting that I end this story with Julia's own words: "I feel like now I have a sense of how to make something happen, how to bring a project to fruition."

References

Aron, L. (2003). The paradoxical place of enactment in psychoanalysis: Introduction. *Psychoanalytic Dialogues*, 13: 5.

Anfam, D. (1990). *Abstract expressionism*. London: Thames and Hudson.

Bass, A. (2009). The mutuality of change and personal growth in analytic relations: Commentary on paper by Lauren Levine. *Psychoanalytic Dialogues*, 19, 4: 463–467.

Bass, A. (2003). "E" enactments in psychoanalysis: Another medium, another message. *Psychoanalytic Dialogues*, 13, 5: 657–675.

Beebe, B. and Lachmann, F. (2002). *Infant research and adult treatment: Co-constructing interactions*. Hillsdale, NJ: The Analytic Press.

Benjamin, J. (1990). Recognition and destruction: An outline of intersubjectivity. *Psychoanalytic Psychology*, 7 (suppl.): 33–47.

Benjamin, J. (2004). Beyond doer and done to: an intersubjective view of thirdness. *Psychoanalytic Quarterly*, 73: 5–46.

Benjamin, J. (2009). A relational psychoanalysis perspective on the necessity of acknowledging failure in order to restore the facilitating and containing features of the intersubjective relationship (the shared third). *International Journal of Psychoanalysis*, 90: 441–450.

Benjamin, J. (2010). Where's the gap and what's the difference? *Contemporary Psychoanalysis*, 46: 112–119.

Bromberg, P.M. (2000). Potholes on the royal road. *Contemporary Psychoanalysis*, 36: 5–28.

Bromberg, P. (2006). *Awakening the dreamer: Clinical journeys*. Mahwah, NJ: The Analytic Press.

Bromberg, P. (1998). *Standing in the spaces: Essays on clinical process, trauma, and dissociation*. Hillsdale, NJ: The Analytic Press.

Csikszentmihalyi, M. (1990). *Flow: The psychology of optimal experience*. New York: Harper Perennial.

Cooper, S. (2000). Mutual containment in the analytic situation. *Psychoanalytic Dialogues*, 10: 169–194.

Cooper, S.H. (2004). State of the hope: The new bad object in the therapeutic action of psychoanalysis. *Psychoanalytic Dialogues*, 14: 527–551.

Davies, J. (2004). Whose bad objects are we anyway? Repetition and our elusive love affair with evil. *Psychoanalytic Dialogues*, 14, 6: 711–732.

Davies, J. (1999). Getting cold feet, defining "safe enough" borders: Dissociation, multiplicity, and integration in the analyst's experience. *Psychoanalytic Quarterly*, LXVIII: 184–208.

Ehrenberg, D. (1992). *The intimate edge*. New York: Norton.

Ehrenberg, D. (1996). On the analyst's emotional availability and vulnerability. *Contemporary Psychoanalysis*, 32: 275–285.

Gallese, V. (2004). "Being like me:" Self-other identity, mirror neurons, and empathy. In S. Hurley and N. Chater, (Eds.) *Perspectives on imitation: From neuroscience to social science*. Boston: MIT Press.

Gallese, V. (2009). Mirror neurons, embodied simulation, and the neural basis of social identification. *Psychoanalytic Dialogues*, 19: 519–536.

Ghent, E. (1992). Paradox and process. *Psychoanalytic Dialogues*, 2: 135–159.

Ghent, E. (1990). Masochism, submission, surrender: Masochism as a perversion of surrender. *Contemporary Psychoanalysis*, 26, 1: 108–135.

Harris, A. (2009). You must remember this. *Psychoanalytic Dialogues*, 19: 2–21.

Hoffman, I. (1998). *Ritual and spontaneity in the psychoanalytic process: A dialectical-constructivist view*. New York: Analytic Press.

Levine, L. (2009a). Transformative aspects of our own analyses and their resonance in our work with our patients. *Psychoanalytic Dialogues*, 19: 454–462.

Levine, L. (2009b). Impasse and resonance across relational realms: Reply to commentaries. *Psychoanalytic Dialogues*, 19: 480–485.

Loewald, H. (1979). The waning of the Oedipus Complex. *Journal of the American Psychoanalytic Association*, 27: 751–775.

Mitchell, S. (1993). *Hope and dread in psychoanalysis*. New York: Basic Books.

Milner, M. (1957). *On not being able to paint*. London: Heineman.

Ogden, T. (2009). *Rediscovering psychoanalysis: Thinking and dreaming, learning and forgetting*. London: Routledge.

Phillips, A. (1988). *Winnicott*. Cambridge: Harvard University Press.

Ringstrom, P. (2012). Commentary on paper by Commentary on Paper by Lauren Levine. *Psychoanalytic Dialogues,* 22, 478–488.

Rosenfeld, H.A. (1987). *Impasse and interpretation*. London: Tavistock.

Schore, A. (2003). *Affect regulation and the repair of the self*. New York: Norton.

Seligman, S. (2009). Temporality and spontaneity in infancy and psychoanalysis. Paper presented at the International Meeting of the International Association of Relational Psychoanalysis and Psychotherapy. Tel Aviv, June.

Slavin & Kriegman (1998). Illusion and uncertainty in psychoanalytic writing. *International Journal of Psychoanalysis*, 79: 333–347.

Stern, D.N., Sander, L., Nahum, J., Harrison, A., Lyons-Ruth, K., Morgan, A., Bruschweiler-Stern, N., and Tronick, E. (1998). Non-interpretative mechanisms in psychoanalytic therapy: The "something more" than interpretation. *International Journal of Psychoanalysis*, 79: 903–921.

Trevarthen, C. (1980). The foundations of intersubjectivity: Development of interpersonal and cooperative understanding in infants. In D.R. Olson (Ed.) *The social foundation of language and thought: Essays in honor of Jerome Bruner* (316–342). New York: Norton.

Winnicott, D.W. (1971). *Playing and reality*. London: Tavistock.

Winnicott, D.W. (1969). The use of an object and relating through identification. In *Playing and reality*. London: Tavistock.

Winnicott, D.W. (1967). Mirror-Role of mother and family in child development. In Playing and reality.

Winnicott, D.W. (1964). *The infant, the child, and the outside world*. Baltimore: Pelican.

Winnicott, D.W. (1958). The capacity to be alone. In *The maturational processes and the facilitating environment*. New York: International Universities Press, 1965.

Chapter 3

Surviving Destruction and Its Creative Potential for Agency and Desire

Barely six months into our work together, Jack rode his bicycle up to the George Washington Bridge and climbed the fence, intending to jump, then re-considered. It was as if he had come into treatment to collapse—to be saved, or not, at the last moment. The image of Jack up on the bridge, on the brink of destruction, was burned into my imagination early on. I felt pushed to the precipice myself, to the edge of my capacity as an analyst, as Jack got deeply into my psyche, under my skin, kept me up at night when he was suicidal. Immersing myself in the depths of his self-loathing and hopelessness was agonizing, and the ongoing fear that he would kill himself, exhausting.

In this chapter, I will explore ways in which a mutual survival of Jack's destructiveness opened potential space for creativity, agency, and desire in both of us. When Jack was acutely suicidal and dissociated, it was an excruciating, and often maddening process for me to bear and help him bear his destructiveness. I will describe how each of us needed to free ourselves from old identifications and constraints, to recognize and mobilize our own capacity for destructiveness and agency and mourn ungrieved losses in order to have the courage to swim together in dangerous, deadly waters. I believe my struggling to hang in there with him in the face of his deadness and deadliness, without retaliating or withdrawing (Ghent, 1992; Winnicott, 1968), helped us both imagine a sense of psychic future (Cooper, 2010; Loewald, 1960) and creative possibility.

Destruction and loss are necessary parts of transformation and growth. Bion (1970) suggests that change is a moment of catastrophe, and that grappling with catastrophic change is an indispensable

DOI: 10.4324/9781003367475-4

aspect of psychic growth (Goldberg, unpublished paper). At the moment of change, you look into the abyss. Imagine Jack up on the Bridge, weighing the binary possibilities of what felt to him like catastrophic change and self-destruction. Jack felt unbearably trapped in his unhappy marriage and strict religion, yet could not envision a way out. Extricating himself from these structures that he had relied upon for identity and stability, his marriage and his faith, felt both necessary for his sense of aliveness, and cataclysmic. Facing a frightening sense of emptiness and fear of the unknown, it was as if Jack had to kill off parts of himself in order to re-build his own sense of internal structure.

The shadow of history also loomed over him and pressed down upon him up on the George Washington Bridge, as Jack was on the verge of repeating with his own children, his father's abandonment 30 years earlier. Yet, unlike his father who had left their family when Jack was four with little contact afterwards, Jack has tried over the years to be a loving, involved father to his own children, even while battling severe depression. He has struggled mightily in the analysis to break a transgenerational cycle of trauma and abandonment by embracing his disavowed rage, becoming aware of and mourning his unconscious identification with his father.

The fantasy of jumping off the George Washington Bridge, a dramatic act, may have felt to Jack, in some respects, like an act of freedom, a reclaiming of power and control. When he felt most despairing, killing himself felt like a desperate desire for change at all cost, a way to free himself from pain without having to face the destructiveness of that act. Jack's telling me about his suicidal fantasies and impulses echoes Winnicott's (1956) notion of the anti-social tendency as a *sign of hope*, a search for a holding environment, "a search for an environmental provision that has been lost." Winnicott suggests that the child's resulting destructiveness is a search for "environmental stability which will stand the strain resulting from impulsive behavior" (p. 310). This has echoes in Jack's history, as well as in our transference-countertransference, embedded in his continual, provocative testing of me and my capacity to contain him.

In our work together, a mutual survival of deadly destructiveness opened the possibility for catastrophic change and creative transformation. Jack has come a long way from that dark moment looking down at the ominous water below; he is building a new life for himself. An architect by profession, he is also a photographer, and recently gave me a gift; a beautiful photograph he took of the inside of the Statue of Liberty, looking up at the interwoven metal beams, the complex internal structure of this towering figure. The photo seems in a sense, like the inverse of the view from the bridge, looking down at the abyss. It reflects layers of internal change that emerged from a tumultuous analytic journey to the depths of despair and back.

This photograph of the tangled metal structure inside the Statue of Liberty holds enormous complexity in terms of the history of our relationship; the ways in which we became entangled with *each other*, and how hard we have worked to put dissociated affect states into words. The photo has a claustrophobic feeling, with no windows and no air to breathe, perhaps reflecting ways in which we had both felt trapped with each other, a mutual sense of entrapment. Immersing myself in the depths of his anguish and hopelessness was harrowing, and entailed living with acute anxiety, powerlessness, and rage. It felt as if we were caught in a sado-masochistic dance, as Jack aggressively used the threat of suicide as power over me, continually testing the limits of my emotional availability.

The photograph also seemed to reflect Jack's fantasies of penetration, of getting inside a woman, inside me. I experienced his fantasies of penetration as both erotic and in terms of Ghent's (1990) reframing of sadism as probing or object finding, the wish to impinge in order to know and be known. Building on Winnicott's (1968) notions of the transformative dimensions of aggression and destructiveness for creative growth, Ghent (1990) writes about probing, attacking, or object finding as a sign of hope, an effort to reach and recognize, to "dis-cover" another. Ghent's iconic notion of surrender entails the longing to be "found, recognized, penetrated to the core so as to become real, or as Winnicott put it ..., 'to come into being'" (p. 122). These notions of probing and object-finding resonate for me in my work with Jack, as his life or death efforts to get me to hold him in mind, hold him inside!, and bear witness to his unbearable pain.

I believe Jack needed me to understand and experience the helplessness, rage, and pervasive sense of shame he had experienced growing up with a depressed, unpredictably angry mother who locked herself in her room for days, an abandoning father, and a step-father who was threatened by and demeaning of Jack's intellectual curiosity and creative pursuits. It took time to metabolize, and to experience in the transference-countertransference, the ways in which he felt tortured and trapped, enraged yet dependent. Jack did not seem to have access to the agentic father who had left his mother, as he seemed identified with the mother who had felt frozen and trapped. I think he needed me to feel the depths of his pain, to not abandon him like his parents when he pushed me to the brink, but to accompany him to the edge of the abyss—without falling in. Jack kept both of us on the brink of mortal danger for what felt like an interminable length of time.

Finally, I received the photograph from Jack as a gift, a token of gratitude for accompanying him on this perilous journey, through dark, unknown waters, for not losing faith in him. We explored the photo as both a creative act and a complex act of reparation. I have deep respect for Jack's resilience, which I think surprised both of us, for his capacity to hit bottom and keep on fighting. No longer trapped alone on the bridge staring down at the depths, Jack now feels more firmly grounded in the present—and can imagine a future. Jack has widened his lens, as the bridge has faded from foreground to background. He can look down the Hudson, see the movement of the currents and the Statue of Liberty on the horizon. The iconic statue in the photograph is a symbol of freedom for immigrants entering new lands.

In the Beginning

In his darkest moments, early in treatment, Jack sat curled up on my couch, dissolved in tears. Lifting his head out of his hands with great effort, he stared at me, a haunting stare that pierced right through me. Jack believed his loneliness in the marriage and their lack of passion reflected something deeply wrong with him. He felt a pervasive sense of shame, and little sense of his own rage, power, or agency. Killing himself felt less frightening than bearing his guilt and responsibility for breaking up his family. He began to question his faith, cursing God for having lived a religious life, which, to him, had entailed huge sacrifices, while still feeling so unhappy and unfulfilled. Jack's religious beliefs had given him a sense of purpose and groundedness, but now it felt as if his faith bound him more tightly and irreparably to a marriage he found stifling. Because his religion dictated that marriage was "forever," leaving his wife and family felt impossible to imagine. We worked on giving himself permission to dream and fantasize, to envision other lives and other possibilities, all of which felt like a revelation to him.

Ogden (2009) describes people unable to dream as "trapped in an endless, unchanging world of what is," (p. 16), and psychoanalysis as a process which "facilitates the patient's dreaming himself into existence" (p. 17). It seemed that Jack felt trapped in an endless, unchanging world of what is, a life that could not be intelligibly lived (Butler, 2009), because of an unmourned past. Mourning had been foreclosed in Jack's family of origin after his father left. The four-year-old boy who had longed for his father went underground as Jack grew up identified with his mother's grief and resentment. As an adolescent in his small, Midwestern, working-class town, he had felt deeply lonely, and constricted by his family's religious strictures. He yearned to be free to have girlfriends and sexual experiences. Now, Jack could not free himself and move on in his life without feeling like a bad man like his father. Suicide felt like the only way to kill off an internalized bad object. This unconscious identification with his father led to his almost abandoning his own children.

Six Months Later

It was a Friday afternoon, the weekend before Thanksgiving. Jack was telling me a story, a story that's lost to me now, buried under the rubble of the devastating disclosure I had not anticipated. Suddenly, he looked at the clock, realizing we are running out of time. "I guess I should tell you what happened last night." Jack told me that late the night before, he had been feeling "really down" leaving work, and could not bear to go home. Instead, he rode his bike up to the George Washington Bridge and began climbing the fence to jump, only changing his mind at the last moment. I felt flooded by a range of feelings: rage, terror, self-doubt. Why hadn't I seen this coming? Why had he waited until now to tell me? Why hadn't he called when he felt suicidal? And, importantly, what made him change his mind and climb down? Warily, ambivalently, I agreed not to hospitalize him, as he promised to check in with me over the weekend and insisted he would not kill himself. I was engulfed by anxiety and dread all weekend.

Was this an unconscious bid for me to feel his sense of entrapment and impotent rage, a desperate projective identification that he needed me to feel, to grasp, to struggle with? A projective identification as communication of his internal state that he needed me to feel from the inside out; an attempt to both destroy me and find me? Echoes of Winnicott and Ghent, here as well.

Just days later, the Wednesday night before Thanksgiving, Jack upped the ante, leaving me a message late at night asking me to call him, a message I did not hear until the next morning. When I called back, Jack told me that he had spent the night locked in his office, lying under his desk, feeling lonely and alone, hoping that I would return his call. He had had a dream, or was it a fantasy? of cutting himself open with a knife, from his neck to his groin. He was horrified, disgusted by what he saw inside; he was filled with worms. I felt terrified—and terrorized—by his threats of violence and self-harm, and haunted by this fantasy, a provocative communication. But, I also heard Jack's message of how exposed he felt in our therapy, like a big open wound. I heard how disgusted and ashamed he felt of his vulnerability and dependency, his concern that I would be disgusted too. But was this fantasy holding some aspect of hope as well as destruction? Hope that that I would hold him in mind over our Thanksgiving break, that I would be able to see and hear his shame and disgust, and not turn away?

These events coincided with the first anniversary of my father's death from a heart attack, a deep and profound loss for me. Still unconsciously identified with a father he had never mourned, perhaps on some level, Jack sensed my increased vulnerability and grief for my own father, a subtle emotional abandonment on my part; fathers' abandonment of sons and daughters. Was there something about my preoccupation with my own father's death that rendered me less available to Jack? His dream/fantasy of cutting himself open cut deeply into me as well, evoking an uncanny association to the open-heart surgeries that had saved my father's life—twice. But, the doctors could not save my father when his heart finally gave out. Could I save Jack?

I had lived with the threat of my father dying since his first bypass surgery at age 42, when I was 16. For all those years, whenever the phone rang late at night, *my* heart stopped—dreading the news of another cardiac emergency. Clearly, the threat of late night emergency phone calls, threatening loss and abandonment, had old, dysregulating reverberations for me. My father had been an intense, dominating figure, loving and generous, but stubbornly determined to live his life without compromise due to his health concerns. While I admired his passion and indomitable spirit, his refusal to abide by his doctor's orders, which bordered on self-destructiveness, made me feel both helpless and enraged. While it had never occurred to me to tell Jack about the anniversary of my father's death, I wonder how much he may have unconsciously sensed my own profound sense of loss, as well as my over-determined fear, anger, and vulnerability, in the face of his self-destructiveness. It was not at all clear to me whether Jack and I would be able to dwell together in our mutual vulnerability; whether my access to my own anger and grief would expand potential space or destroy it.

Relentlessly, Jack and I tried to understand what triggered his shifts from depression to suicidality. His shifts in self-states felt jarring and mysterious, to him and to me. He was *in* one state, then *in* another with little capacity for self-reflection. I told him that it was hard for him to keep in mind that he did not always feel this way, that self-states shift, do not last forever, that there were times when he felt more engaged and optimistic. I said, "These are the parts of you that stop you from acting when you feel suicidal, the self-protective parts, the parts of you that made you decide to climb down from the bridge instead of jumping."

Perhaps, I was also evoking the parts of my father that had kept him going for so long with a serious heart condition. Though he did not always take care of himself, he was fiercely determined to survive. I told Jack more than once that killing himself would devastate his children, and dramatically increase the chances of their committing suicide. Perhaps this was an aggressive act on my part, standing up to his self-destructive self-state, appealing to the loving and responsible part of him, just as I had, over a lifetime, with my father. But, the loving, responsible part of Jack was so split-off from the despairing, self-destructive part, that he felt my continuing to hold his children in mind was akin to "dropping" him. He became enraged with me, told me I was just making him feel guiltier. I responded, "Guilt's not necessarily a bad thing ... But there's a difference between guilt and responsibility, and you aren't owning the destructiveness of this act." This feels reminiscent of Mitchell's (2000) distinction between guilt and guiltiness. Mitchell suggests that guilt entails a sense of painful growth and shared vulnerability, holding ourselves accountable for our culpability without self-pity, while guiltiness involves a sense of victimization and subtle interpersonal coercion.

Jack questioned my honesty and reliability, told me I was hurting him, lying to him, not available in the ways he needed me to be. He left desperate, angry messages on my machine as the gaps between our three sessions a week felt interminable. He told me, "I feel lonely and fucked up that I'm so dependent on you, that you're the person I'm closest to. You're my lifeline and I'm just one of your patients." As hard as I tried, inevitably I failed him, again and again. I had a powerful sense of how he must have felt trying to save his depressed, angry mother locked in her room, his dread of her deadness and deadliness, terrified that she would kill herself, that he would not be able to save her. Echoes of the "Dead Mother" (Green, 1986), described by Gerson (2009) as "an absent presence whose effect on the child is like that of a black hole that relentlessly sucks the child's vitality ... Her emptiness becomes his, and his becomes the task to fill them both, to create presence in the space left by absence" (p. 354). I felt like I was in quicksand, that all my efforts were useless or ineffective. I knew I was feeling too responsible and controlled by Jack, but I could not seem to stabilize myself or him. The countertransference demands on me were reaching a breaking point.

Then I had a dream about my father.

I was in the kitchen of my childhood apartment in New York City. Suddenly my father was there with me. In the dream, I was aware that he had died, and was elated to see him alive. In disbelief, I went to hug him. I felt enormously grateful to be able to see him and hug him and feel him hugging me. Then, as I was pondering the impossibility and wishfulness of this encounter, my father collapsed in my arms. I was devastated, losing him once again.

Was this an unconscious effort to dream my father back into existence, as I was desperately struggling to enliven the psychically dead man in front of me? Could I keep Jack from collapsing in my arms? Or, alternatively, was I having trouble allowing him to collapse in my arms, defending against a necessary, and mutual surrender? (Ghent, 1990)

Consulting with a colleague (Lisa Lyons, personal communication, February, 2006) helped me gain perspective, feel more grounded, and regain a sense of my own power and agency. I was deeply appreciative, as our conversation helped me break out of a state of aloneness and collapse, freeing me to find my own words to address the impasse with Jack directly, to be able to verbalize in a way that Jack could hear, what I had been experiencing on an embodied yet unformulated level (Stern, 1997, 2010).

I told him I felt like he was holding a gun to my head, that I could not help him, and be fully present with him, if I felt so terrorized by his self-destructiveness. I told him that he needed to promise not to kill himself for a year, to give us time and space to work together; that we were exploring some very deep, shameful parts of himself in order to understand the pain underlying his suicidality, and we needed to be able trust each other, to work together. Jack seemed intrigued, curious, and comforted that I seemed to recognize that he "had likeable parts too." In this session, perhaps I felt more like a new, sturdy, non-collapsing mother. I was communicating that I would not abandon him in his most despairing self-states, but that he needed to join me, to take more responsibility for his actions and their destructive consequences.

I believe this communication served multiple functions. In sharing my countertransference with Jack, I was making him aware of my own subjectivity and emotional limits, as well as my vulnerability and capacity to be deeply affected by him. I was also signifying that I had faith in his ability to keep himself alive, that I was willing to hang in there with him, but only if he were a willing partner, prepared to own his own power. I was communicating that the state he was in was foreclosing his creativity and agency as well as mine. My interpretation had a freeing impact on me too, as I felt relieved, stronger, and less stuck; freer to access my own inner resources and to remind Jack of his. He said, "A year feels like a long time to keep fighting to stay alive." But we kept talking, and our dialogue ushered in a calmer period that felt more mutual and engaged. In retrospect, I think the metaphor of his "holding a gun to my head" reflected my increasing capacity to symbolize and metabolize Jack's and my own aggression and power.

I believe the holding from my colleague, when I was feeling destabilized and overwhelmed, was crucial to my being able to hold Jack. The consultation seems to me to have been a kind of parallel process, as my feeling held in mind and grounded by my colleague allowed me to serve a more containing, integrative function for Jack. My standing up to him was reassuring for both of us, a sign of my resilience and renewed capacity to withstand his ruthlessness, which would be continue to be tested for months to come. I went from allowing Jack to hold me hostage to rediscovering my own power and agency.

Perhaps my dream about my father played a role here as well, capturing something crucial about the link between destruction and transformation. In the dream, I dreamt my father both into and out of existence, as he was re-enlivened and then collapsed again in my arms. My father had been a loving, but complicated and challenging man, who held enormous power in our family. In some ways, I had felt held hostage by him too, less able to own my own power in the face of his dominating presence, which made me more vulnerable to enacting that dynamic with Jack. The consultation helped me gain access to more adult parts of myself, to move out of a younger, more helpless self-state. In this way, my own history intertwines with Jack's, as the process of mourning my father entailed disentangling old, limiting identifications. As devastated as I felt about losing my father, was there also something I needed to destroy in my relationship with him that freed me, and freed me to stand up to Jack? This is reminiscent of Loewald's (1979) parricide, the killing off of parental authority, in order to find one's unique voice, one's power and creativity. But there is more. In Loewald's model of separation and emancipation, there is also internalization and identification. Perhaps in the holding from my father, and the mourning of my father, I was internalizing a parent who could be both tough and loving, strengthening me so that I would be able to hold Jack.

As I wrote in chapter one,

> As psychoanalysts, our own relational stories, our "wounds that must serve as tools" (Harris, 2009) represent both our greatest

liabilities and potential for change, at times facilitating and at times impeding our capacity to engage deeply in the analytic process.

(Levine, 2009)

Harris (2009) reminds us that negotiating impasse often entails a process of mourning on the analyst's part, a necessary grieving of the analyst's "wounds that must serve as tools," in order to restore clinical momentum and create the potential for change (p. 5).

A Spark of Aliveness: The Emergence of The Erotic

An emerging erotic transference felt like a sign of hope, a spark of aliveness, a search for jouissance. With some trepidation, Jack allowed himself to fantasize, to imagine feeling loved and desired. I felt profoundly moved by this deepening of attachment and excited by the erotic aliveness in the analytic space, by Jack's willingness to risk sharing his fantasies about me and with me. This allowed me to get to know him as the man he could be, and allowed him to see himself reflected through my eyes. The treatment felt enlivened, passionate, open to possibility. But after a while, trying to hold longing and desire in the realm of fantasy became excruciating for Jack. He angrily accused me of seduction and betrayal, as the asymmetry of our relationship felt intolerable, enraging. He told me *his* fantasies; why wouldn't I tell him *mine*? I considered his provocative, yet understandable question and struggled with how to talk with him about the man I was coming to know without being overly seductive. I felt the fragile potential space we had built together collapsing around us. It felt like a huge loss, I'm sure for both of us. Just as Jack felt that his wife's sexual unresponsiveness reflected something deeply flawed and undesirable in him, my holding the boundaries, and the asymmetry of our therapeutic relationship felt shaming, humiliating. Perhaps our talking about erotic desire and the feelings that mobilized in him had felt too threatening in the context of his deep vulnerability.

As Jack was becoming more enlivened and in touch with his own desire, he began to have sex with his wife, who was trying desperately to convince him to stay in the marriage. Although Jack appreciated her efforts and was glad to be having sex again, it felt like too little, too late. Then, although they were using condoms, according to Jack, Maggie became pregnant with a fourth child and refused to terminate the pregnancy. Jack could not bear to explore his part in the pregnancy. My efforts to open up his active involvement in the pregnancy were met with anger and withdrawal. Feeling utterly stuck and hopeless, Jack plummeted into despair and became actively suicidal. This time, his psychiatrist and I decided to hospitalize him. The line between aliveness and deadness, procreativity and destructiveness felt porous and precarious. Jack seemed thankful for the hospital's containment. Me too! The hospital served a containing function for both of us. His weeklong hospitalization was traumatic but mobilizing, jolting him into the realization that he was not as bad off as the psychotic patients around him.

In our first session back, Jack told me that the day he came home from the hospital, his children tackled him and "buried him under a pile of hugs." The striking irony of Jack being "buried" under his children's hugs was not lost on us. It seemed to capture the ways in which his deep love for his children could paradoxically exist side by side with his desolation and suicidal impulses; the first signs of his nascent capacity to create links between self-states. Although I did not share my dream about hugging my father with Jack, being buried under a pile of hugs also had reverberations for me in my dream as I felt held, and then abandoned by my father's dying again in my arms. Jack described how profound it felt to him to be hugged and held by his children, reminded of their love and attachment, which he had dissociated in his most suicidal self-states. I understood this on a deep, embodied level. Over the next few months, Jack began to feel stronger and more stable, but this process was far from linear, with periods of profound depression and provocative suicidal threats.

Eight months later, their new baby was born and Jack became intensely attached, taking a four-week paternity leave from work to spend time with him. Though he knew a separation from his wife was inevitable, he now felt less anxious, more patient. He brought his three-week-old son to our session, and I was immediately struck by how utterly comfortable he seemed as a father, moved by this new life he had created. He asked if I wanted to hold the baby, then expertly swaddled him and placed him gently in my arms. I felt a powerful sensory experience of Jack's connection to this child, of his capacity to care for him, of his wanting me to feel it, too. Having come through the eye of the storm together, to the other side—back to life, I couldn't help wondering, "Whose baby was this anyway?" I felt a keen awareness of how far he had traveled from desired/repudiated pregnancy to much loved son. We talked about the multiple layers of meaning of this new life, and of Jack's handing him to me to hold, how this baby no longer felt like an obstacle to Jack's imagining a future for himself. We talked about the erotic transference as birthing hope for a new connection and a life beyond despair.

Endings and New Beginnings

A few months later, Jack's mother became seriously ill. He spent her last weeks caring for her in the hospital, feeding her, painting her toenails, saying goodbye. Worlds away from his adolescence when she had locked herself in her room, inaccessible and depressed for days, holding him hostage, his mother now allowed him to care for her intimately as she lay dying. Jack could now take the risk to reach out to her with tenderness and compassion. A reparative mourning process. Immediately after his mother died, and without conscious forethought, Jack contacted his father for the first time in 21 years to inform him of her death. This was a very striking, spontaneous act that took me by surprise; Jack did not tell me about it until afterward. The death of one parent opened the possibility of reconnection with the other.

What freed Jack in his mother's death? Separating from his mother entailed the destruction of old family structure, allowing for the creation of the new. In reaching out to his father, Jack took a huge emotional risk, which he now felt free to take for the first time. This courageous act had deep resonance in the leap of faith we had both taken in our work together; the risk of deep mutual vulnerability. To Jack's great surprise, his father replied that evening; a warm, engaging email, opening a new dialogue. This stimulated a host of complicated reactions involving anger and grief that we processed over many months, a search for lost time, lost fathers and mothers, mourning the loss of the person he could have become. But, Jack was also anxious to get to know his father from an adult perspective, with more depth, texture, and generosity. In the process of getting to know him, Jack discovered that his father was a photographer too.

Breaking the intergenerational transmission of trauma, of fathers abandoning children, demanded that Jack mourn unconscious identifications with both parents, coming to terms with the ways in which his mother had also abandoned him through her depression and unpredictable rages. Through our work, his father became more human, less of an icon, opening the possibility of leaving his own marriage without feeling like a bad man, but instead, a man who wanted to be more fully alive. This dysregulating, re-configuring of old object ties, the re-writing of the family narrative, seemed to open psychic space, enabling Jack to move toward separation in a very different, more hopeful state of mind.

Jack separated from Maggie with a mixture of dread and exhilaration, a challenge that entailed managing his guilt over his newfound excitement and desire and the necessary destruction that that entailed. I had to manage my own anxiety and dread about Jack leaving a wife who had taken care of him, perhaps held him together in many ways, even though the relationship had been unsatisfying. How would he manage on his own? How would he, or rather *we,* manage without Maggie? Jack was eager to explore the adolescence he had longed for and never had. Tolerating loneliness and solitude was difficult; he threw himself into dating with manic abandon. Jack was intoxicated by the thrill of seducing and being seduced—the mutual flirtation, the first kiss, a newfound capacity to give women multiple orgasms.

When Jack was first dating, I was aware of his efforts to get to know me, anew; different parts of me, more intimately through the various women he went out with. He dated several Jewish women, psychologists or psychiatrists, runners like me, even a woman named Lauren. Telling me about his dates and sexual experiences in intimate detail felt like part of that effort. At times, he sought my admiration and recognition for his sexual prowess; often he tried to titillate me with his romantic adventures. We talked about the different ways in which Jack wanted me to experience his sexual awakening. I was acutely aware of the ways in which his newfound freedom and sense of himself as attractive and desirable to women felt crucial and deeply enlivening. This felt poignant to me, and I resonated with Jack's excitement and sense of adventure. It felt like the stirring of longing and desire was now less likely to become conflated with abandonment and shame, as Jack felt more hopeful and alive. Rejection by women felt devastating at first, but over time, Jack is learning to manage it with grace and perspective. He has now had several long-term relationships.

Separating from his marriage and his faith, destroying the two main structures that had bound him, in both senses of the word, left Jack feeling destabilized and unmoored. This took great courage, a willingness to mourn, to wrestle with, what felt like catastrophic change (Bion, 1970), a crucial aspect of psychic growth. Goldberg (unpublished paper), drawing on Bion, suggests, "The way to live in a catastrophically changing world is to become adept in the ways of catastrophic change. In analysis, this involves the emotional experience of making (and losing and re-making) meaning." Goldberg writes "that Bion's insight about catastrophic change, elaborated by Ogden (2004, 2009) and Ferro (2008), is that it is the presence of the other—the dream-like reverie of another mind—that allows one's own dreaming to proceed" (p. 3).

A Dream

Then Jack had a dream evocative of Bion's notion of change as a moment of catastrophe, which I believe captures his increasing capacity to embrace previously disowned aggression and use destructiveness creatively. In the dream, Jack looked up at "old-fashioned elevated train tracks from another era," showing me with his hand the shape of a "beautiful arched structure above the tracks." Suddenly there was an earthquake; the destruction was "spectacular." The tracks came crashing down; yet somehow it was clear that no one was hurt. Jack was with his son and they went underground down steps damaged by the earthquake. An older man kidnapped his son and Jack chased him through tunnels, finally catching him, and beat him up. Maggie and his other children were there now, looking for a way to get out from underground. Maggie said that she was going to look for a way out with one of the kids and left Jack with the others. Jack was angry with her for separating the family. Finally, they found a way out and Jack yelled at her for making bad decisions and putting the kids at risk.

This powerful dream seemed to reflect a central aspect of the treatment, a mutual surviving of destruction of external and internal structures that somehow we both survived. This "spectacular" destruction entailed tearing down the main structures that had both held and bound Jack throughout his life, his marriage and his faith, in order to free himself to live the life he desired as he grew and changed. In our early years together, the guilt had felt like too much to bear; self-destruction had felt like the only way out. In retrospect, perhaps the dream holds countertransference as well as transference narrative threads, as the process of mourning my father, which entailed the destruction of old, constricting identifications freed me to access my own power and aggression, and to encourage and embrace Jack's agency and desire (Levine, 2009). The dream seems to capture Jack's awareness of the precariousness of our analytic journey, the vulnerability and risk for both of us, and the courage to go to deep places in himself, and with me. It reflects his increasing capacity to move more fluidly between self-states, rather than being stuck in despair, as well as his evolving capacity to mobilize his aggression in the service of agency and desire, including challenging me and getting angry with me more directly. We considered all this and more, the multiple meanings of the dream, including Jack's embracing of previously disowned anger at Maggie for her part in the marriage's demise, instead of continuing to blame himself alone. A striking shift from his earlier tendency to internalize rage, leading to collapse and self-destructive impulses.

Another strand in the dream is Jack's guilt over the pain he caused his family, guilt that he had not been able to access earlier in the treatment when he was acutely suicidal and dissociated. We talked about how bearing his own destructiveness and guilt for wanting more was an ongoing challenge. In beating up the older man, who Jack associated to his father, he was expressing his anger toward his father for "kidnapping" him, holding him hostage, both in his identification with his father as a "bad man," and by keeping him stuck in the role of an abandoned little boy. In beating up the kipnapper, Jack was protecting his own children, breaking the intergenerational repetition of abandonment; fathers rescuing instead of abandoning.

Discussion

What was mutative in the analysis? How did destructiveness that at first appeared deadly become a source of agency, passion, and creative change for both of us? As I wrote in chapter 1, on transformative aspects of our own analyses and their resonance in our work with our patients,

> when it goes well, psychoanalysis gives one the experience of being in a relationship that feels safe enough, as Harris (2009) suggests, "to open access to unbearable affects," so that one can begin to feel less ashamed and humiliated of those split-off, unacceptable parts of oneself.

But the analyst needs to be able to embrace and bear those damaging introjects which interweave and collide with her own ungrieved losses and those of her patients without falling apart herself, in order for therapeutic movement and psychic change to occur (Harris, 2009; Levine, 2012; McLaughlin, 2006).

A pivotal moment occurred when I reached a breaking point and found my own voice through the consultation with my colleague. I experienced an important countertransferential shift from standing on the edge, trying to pull Jack out of the abyss to a willingness to go there with him, to not abandon him as long as he agreed to stay alive, to work with me. In retrospect, I can appreciate the ways in which I did abandon him on some level, when he was at his most suicidal. It had felt too frightening to join him in his despair because of my fear of his impulsivity and dissociation, as well as my vulnerability to feeling held hostage. As I wondered after my dream about my father, "Had I been having trouble allowing Jack to collapse in my arms, defending against a necessary, mutual surrender?" (Ghent, 1990). It was not until I experienced the grounding and support from my colleague that I felt strong enough to trust myself and Jack to live through his anguish, to walk around together in the abyss. This required a leap of faith on both our parts, a surrender to a deeper level of intimacy.

I began my work with Jack in a year of mourning my own father's death, and could not have anticipated the ways in which my vulnerability to my own grief would have powerful reverberations in our work together – how it would shape my own listening and counter-transference as both grieving daughter and the mother of two sons. What Bass (2001) calls the mutuality of vulnerability. I could not have anticipated the ways in which a mutual survival of destructiveness and shared vulnerability would open potential space for Jack to mourn his parents, his religion, and the life he had built in order to make room for desire, creativity, and growth. Perhaps he had needed to hit bottom, again and again, to destroy the old constricting structures he had built in order to feel freer to choose the life he desired. Although I have focused more in this chapter on the challenges of separating from his wife without abandoning his children like his father, leaving his religion also shook Jack to the core. Over the years, Jack has taught me, his Jewish analyst, a lot about the richness and complexity of the religion in which he was raised. Leaving his church entailed a huge loss of identity, spirituality, and community.

It has now been 12 years since Jack separated from Maggie. They have developed a strikingly collaborative co-parenting relationship, surely a testament to her resilience, patience, and capacity for forgiveness as well. Jack spends two weeknights and half the weekend with his children. Parenting them has been reparative; a source of pride and generativity. As his children have grown, Jack has given them the message to follow their dreams and passions. I can hear and feel the ways in which Jack has brought to bear his experience of being in analysis in his parenting; ways in which he listens and empathizes with his children and helps them resolve conflicts, recognizing their unique strengths and vulnerabilities. He has a wonderful ability to defuse his children's anger, often with humor, and can set limits while empathizing with their frustration.

Early in our work together, Jack tended to give up, give in, submit in the face of conflict, both between himself and others, and more dangerously, shutting down and becoming self-destructive in the face of internal turmoil. In the transference, Jack completely disavowed anger at me, withdrawing or acting out or being passive-aggressive with little awareness of his rage. Over time, he has become more expressive of his anger toward me, Maggie, his children, and girl-friends. Jack lets me know directly when he feels misunderstood or criticized, or overly challenged by me when he feels too vulnerable.

As he has been able to own his aggression and bear the guilt of his own destructiveness, including breaking his family apart, Jack has become less self-destructive, more aware of his own power and agency.

Though Jack continues to struggle with depression, I don't worry about the bottom falling out. Much less dissociated, he is less likely to feel trapped in any one self-state, and has a firmer sense that self-states shift, will not last forever. In analysis, he and I can more easily shift between states of deep mutual reflection, playfulness, and humor. Instead of collapsing and becoming self-destructive in the face of unbearable turmoil, Jack can increasingly tolerate aggression and loss, and in fact, transform it into art. I sensed intuitively, early on, that nurturing his artistic abilities was critical to his developing a sense of authorship in order to reinvent himself, perhaps even a matter of life or death. Having relied on women for affirmation and self-esteem, creative pursuits, especially photography have become a source of agency, and a way of taking care of himself. Jack has now gotten significant recognition for his photography. In fact, he was recently asked to be the photographer-in-residence at a performance space and is often hired to photograph concerts and dance performances.

Writing about patients is complicated business, full of pitfalls and liabilities. But it holds the potential to deepen and enrich the work in the context of an ongoing treatment, to serve as another level of reflection, supervision and working through. Writing this paper has been a way of taking care of myself and my ongoing relationship with Jack. It came out of a desire to understand how close Jack and I came to the brink of destruction, and to explore how metabolizing destructiveness became a source of aliveness and creative potential, for us both.

And so, I return to the photograph that Jack gave me of the inside of the Statue of Liberty, a picture he took just after the statue had undergone a major renovation. Presumably, the statue is now sturdier, able to weather violent storms as well as internal exploration. In giving me this photograph, perhaps Jack was communicating unconsciously the significance of my allowing him to get deeply inside me, to become acutely unsettled and deeply attached, to know and be known by him. And yet. Jack was also telling me, in this photograph of the tangled metal beams supporting this sculpture, about the non-linearity, the ongoing complexity of growth and change. Looking back at our years together, I am awed by how close we came to the edge of destruction, by the precariousness of a past that almost foreclosed a future, by how much we survived and created together.

References

Bass, A. (2001). It takes one to know one; Or whose unconscious is it anyway? *Psychoanalytic Dialogues*, 11: 683–702.

Bion, W. (1970). *Attention and interpretation*. London: Maresfield Library, 1984.

Butler, J. (2009). *Frames of war: When is life grievable?* London: Verso.

Cooper, S. (2010). *A disturbance in the field: Essays in transference-countertransference engagement*. New York: Routledge.

Gerson, S. (2009). When the third is dead: Memory, mourning, and witnessing in the aftermath of the Holocaust. In *Relational Psychoanalysis*, Vol. 4: Expansion of theory, pp. 347–366.

Ghent, E. (1990). Masochism, submission, surrender: Masochism as a perversion of surrender. *Contemporary Psychoanalysis*, 26, 1: 108–135.

Ghent, E. (1992). Paradox and process. *Psychoanalytic Dialogues*, 2: 135–159.

Goldberg, P. Catastrophic change, communal dreaming, and the counter-catastrophic personality. Unpublished paper.

Green, A. (1986). The dead mother. In *On private madness*. London: Rebuz Press.

Harris, A. (2009). You must remember this. *Psychoanalytic Dialogues*, 19: 2–21.

Levine, L. (2009). Transformative aspects of our own analyses and their resonance in our work with our patients. *Psychoanalytic Dialogues*, 19, 454–462.

Levine, L. (2012). Into thin air: The co-construction of shame, recognition, and creativity in an analytic process. *Psychoanalytic Dialogues*, 22: 456–471.

Loewald, H. (1960). On the therapeutic action of psychoanalysis. *International Journal of Psychoanalysis*, 41: 16–33.

Loewald, H. (1979). The waning of the Oedipus complex. *Journal of the American Psychoanalytic Association*, 27: 751–775.

McLaughlin, J. (2006). *The healer's bent*. Hillsdale, NJ: The Analytic Press.

Mitchell, S. (2000). You've got to suffer if you want to sing the blues: Psychoanalytic reflections on guilt and self-pity. *Psychoanalytic Dialogues*, 10: 713–733.

Ogden, T. (2009). *Rediscovering psychoanalysis: Thinking and dreaming, learning and forgetting*. London: Routledge.

Stern, D.B. (1997). *Unformulated experience: From dissociation to imagination in psychoanalysis.* Hillsdale, NJ: The Analytic press.

Stern, D.B. (2010). *Partners in thought: Working with unformulated experience, dissociation, and enactment.* New York: Routledge.

Winnicott, D.W. (1956). The anti-social tendency. In *Collected papers: Through paediatrics to psychoanalysis.* New York: Basic Books, 1958.

Winnicott, D.W. (1968). The use of an object and relating through identifications. In *Playing and Reality.* London: Tavistock, 1971.

Chapter 4

Mutual Vulnerability: Destruction and Reparation

Twelve years into our work together, after an extended summer break, Lisa tells me, matter-of-factly, "I didn't miss you at all this summer." We lose each other, and find each other, and hurt each other. Over and over. We remember, and dissociate, intimate, agonizing moments, exploring the rapes she endured as a teenager in horrific detail. A mutually inductive amnesia. Our attachment feels powerful and deep; yet, echoing her traumatic past, the ground beneath us can shift seismically without warning. The Other becomes alien or destructive as we shift roles abruptly, unpredictably, from perpetrator to victim to frozen bystander, jarred and destabilized by the affective state of the other.

In the beginning, Lisa's traumatized past was frozen in time, buried in the past. She referred to "Old Lisa" and "New Lisa." It took years of analysis for her to feel safe enough to open the door to Old Lisa, to allow us both to get to know her. The doors open and close. Lisa remembers, and dissociates, the ongoing attachment trauma that infused her relational template, her parents' destructive narcissism, neglect, and psychic violence. Though Lisa had always considered her enmeshed relationship with her mother to be "close," we came to understand her mother's "appropriation and intrusion" (Faimberg, 2005), as depriving Lisa of a mind of her own, leaving her feeling empty and overwhelmed. Building on Bromberg, Lyon et al. (2012) suggest, "Unmetabolized trauma cannot be mentalized, and therefore cannot be mourned. The shards of such ungrieved loss mark the fault lines or vulnerabilities that we carry with us into future relational exchanges." I imagine Lisa and I picking up the shattered pieces,

DOI: 10.4324/9781003367475-5

gathering the intergenerational shards. They cut and injure us both in the process, as my own fault lines and vulnerabilities collide with Lisa's in unpredictable, often disturbing ways.

In this chapter, I will explore the challenges of mutual vulnerability, highlighting psychic collisions in my work with Lisa, a mutual survival of destructiveness and shame, and a reaching toward reparation and mutual recognition. And love. I will describe how mutual vulnerability entails a willingness to be deeply unsettled and dys-regulated by our most wounded and traumatized patients (Harris, 2009). As Ferro (2005) suggests, the courage to engage deeply in psychoanalysis involves abandoning "our state of impermeability and becoming available for assumption and 'contagion'" (p. 67).

Riffing on the Italian playwright, Pirandello's existentialist play, *Six Characters in Search of an Author*, Ferro posits that the mind of the analyst and the mind of the patient, like two authors, work together to communicate what is happening at the depths of the relational exchange. Analyst and patient strive to create a meaningful dialogue that integrates past and present, in the *here and now*. Ghosts from the intergenerational histories of both analyst and patient enter and exit the analytic stage, and the analyst must creatively engage with the multiple characters that emerge in the relational field. Bion suggests, "It takes two minds to think one's most disturbing thoughts." But allowing the other to enter one's most private, shame-filled spaces when one has been deeply violated, takes tremendous courage. For the analyst, finding ways of witnessing without co-opting, knowing without colonizing (Levinas, 1969), can be daunting.

I want to further ground this conversation in Bleger's (1967) notion of the setting, "the totality of phenomena included in the therapeutic relationship between the analyst and the patient" (p. 1), and the Baranger's (2008) ideas of the analytic situation as a dynamic field, in which "two persons remain unavoidably connected and complementary; ... (so that) neither member of the couple can be understood without the other" (p. 796). This dynamic field includes elements of the frame, aspects of time and space, but also, and most relevant to my paper, the intersecting of two subjectivities—two family and sociocultural histories. For the analyst, this bi-personal field includes the analyst's professional her-story, the voices of her own analyst, supervisors, and theoretical forbearers. Furthermore, past and current experiences with other patients reside, often unconsciously or preconsciously in the analyst, emerging unbidden in reveries, dreams and associations, and creating unanticipated opportunities—and enactments—in our work with patients.

As I will describe, I had a terrifying nightmare in the process of writing this paper, which reflected both powerful countertransferential aspects of my work with Lisa, as well as resonance from another harrowing treatment, my work with Jack, about whom I was also writing at the time. Even more destabilizing, my dream contained fears of traumatic loss and abandonment of my own semi-grown children. Mutual vulnerability involves openness to reverberations across manifold relational realms (Bass, 2001; Levine, 2009b, Levine, 2016). It necessitates an essential porousness, an openness to being deeply affected that is an additional burden, a *hazard* of working relationally. As Harris has suggested, we need to be thinking more, and theorizing more, about how we take care of ourselves, as analysts, when we are working in such deep, mutual, and potentially destabilizing ways.

In his fierce commitment to reach his most traumatized patients, those considered "unanalyzable" by standard psychoanalytic technique, Ferenczi developed the radical model of mutual analysis. His courageous experiment entailed huge risks for the analyst, an openness to her own subjectivity and vulnerability, and a willingness to let herself be known by her patients. The publication of Ferenzci's diaries in 1988 revealed the earliest roots of a Relational model of psychoanalysis. Ferenzci recognized both the liability and creative potential of the "dialogue of unconsciouses," between analyst and patient (Bass, 2001; Ferenczi, 1932; Harris 2009). Ferenzci leaned into the problem, and the resource, of the analyst's unconscious and countertransference, the inevitability of enactments, and the importance of collaborative efforts to restore intersubjective relatedness.

A word here about differentiating mutual vulnerability from mutual analysis. The problematic aspects of Ferenczi's forays into mutual analysis are well-known, and reflected on poignantly by Ferenczi himself. In his model, he and his analysands took turns being in the role of the patient, as Ferenczi, challenged by Elizabeth Severn (RN), came to believe that the analyst's unconscious created blind-spots that the patient could perceive and bring to light for mutual exploration and understanding. The notion of mutual vulnerability builds on and indeed deepens Ferenczi's efforts to open the analytic field to the intersubjectivity of both analyst and patient, to the dialogue of unconsciouses, while maintaining the asymmetrical nature of the analytic relationship (Aron, 1996), and a focus on the patient and her concerns.

Lisa and I

Early in treatment, Lisa referred to her traumatized past as Old Lisa, a not-me life, filled with disavowed violence and profound neglect. Over time, we found it lurking in subterranean realms, in her dreams, fantasies, preoccupations: mothers who murder, or let their children drown. In analysis, intimacy and rape get conflated and collapsed. The line between closeness and intrusion feels precarious, carrying the threat of violation for us both. "I didn't miss you at all this summer," says Lisa. Reverberations in multiple registers, multiple realms. Echoes of her parents' destructive narcissism and neglect, a reminder of feeling discarded, erased.

Lisa originally consulted me late in her pregnancy with her second child. Worried that she could not possibly love her second son as much as her first, a not uncommon fear, Lisa in fact, had great difficulty bonding with her second child. This presenting problem, the fear of not bonding with her son, was a dark premonition, and seemed in a sense, an as yet unarticulated fear of the intergenerational transmission of trauma, of not wanting to replicate the damage of the malignant narcissism of her parents with her own children. It also foreshadowed the challenges of linking (Bion, 1959) in the treatment, the complexity of presence and absence, attachment and abandonment, which would characterize our transference-countertransference over time. As Lyon et al. (2012) suggest, "The inability to link ... is the hallmark of the unbearable."

It took years of work together for Lisa to be able to tell me, with full affective force, about the rapes she had endured in early adolescence. Raped at age 12 by her mother's boyfriend, a man whom she had loved and trusted, Lisa was not clear whether her mother was more upset about her being raped, or about having to break up with her boyfriend. As her analyst (and as a mother), when I heard this story about her being raped at such a young age and her mother's excruciatingly narcissistic reaction, it felt almost impossible to bear.

Imagining Lisa being doubly traumatized, first by the rape by a trusted father figure, and then betrayed by her mother's response felt both enraging and heartbreaking. When she was raped a second time at age 13 by her father's colleague, her father did not believe her, so her experience was once again violently disconfirmed by a parental attachment figure. Not surprisingly, Lisa went into a tailspin soon afterward, engaging in promiscuous sex and anaesthetizing herself in a drug-induced haze throughout adolescence.

Years ago, after an intense session in which we were exploring the rapes in agonizing detail, Lisa had a dream. She had read a gruesome story in the *New York Times* that had captured the public's attention, about a mother who had driven her car into a lake, killing herself and three of her children. A fourth child escaped out the window. In her dream, Lisa is standing in shallow water, trying to scream for help, but cannot. There is an enormous wave coming at her. She is terrified of drowning, of being overtaken by the wave. Finally, she yells, "Help me!" out loud, waking herself up. Multiple reverberations of a mother who drowns her children. Rage at her mother, at her father, who didn't protect her, didn't believe her, and the terror of her own identification with the aggressor, and her own aggressive fantasies as a mother. She imagines the rapist: a huge wave overtaking her, pulling her under. The horror in recalling, re-experiencing the rapes with me, the fear of feeling trapped in the analytic car together. To whom is Lisa yelling for help? In analysis, helping is fraught with vulnerability, as I am alternately, unpredictably seen by her as holding, or violating. How do you yell for help when you cannot trust someone to hear your cries, to not abandon you or violate you further? Her parents' discounting, disavowing of her rapes was doubly traumatizing, as they were unwitnessed and unmourned, making intimacy and trust enormously challenging.

For years, Lisa has been haunted by a recurring fantasy in waking life, another watery nightmare. She is standing on the side of a pool, and one of her children falls in. She is frozen. Does not, cannot, jump in to save him. Lisa is horrified by this recurring fantasy, terrified that she would not have the wherewithal to save her child. We have deconstructed this as both an identification with her parents who did not protect her; in fact *put her in harm's way*, and a manifestation of her own post-traumatic, "frozen" response to intergenerational trauma. Who gets rescued or abandoned? Is she the murderous mother, frozen mother or drowning child? In analysis, can Lisa take the risk of jumping in, swimming in these dangerous waters together? *Can I?* Unlike her ocean dream with annihilating waves, a pool is contained, with edges and a frame. But she–and I–can still drown in a pool.

These dreams serve as commentary about where we have been and where we need to go, about how Lisa needs to use me in the Winnicottian sense, whom I need to be for her, and what must be done to me. Mutual vulnerability entails the risk of being dysregulated, haunted by Lisa's traumatic memories and nightmares; projective identification as unconscious communication of Lisa's intolerable, split-off and dissociated self-states. Which leads me to a terrifying dream that I had in the process of writing this paper.

I am in a car with my husband and close friends, in the passenger seat, while my husband is driving. We're all talking and laughing. Suddenly we're careening off a bridge toward the water below, knowing we are going to die. Absolutely panicked about leaving my two sons with no parents, I desperately try to envision ways of escaping from the car, in the air, when it hits the water, when we submerge in the water, even while knowing it's likely impossible. I'm desperate! and refuse to accept drowning and abandoning my kids. In my dream, I am the drowning, traumatized child, the child who escapes out the car window, the mother fighting to not abandon my kids. Fighting for my life. And theirs.

I want to look at this dream of mine from multiple perspectives. Ferro (2006), building on Bion, suggests that the analyst constantly receives, metabolizes, and transforms the patient's verbal and non-verbal stimuli into ongoing reverie, and that the patient's and analyst's psychic collisions create a bi-personal analytic field that is perpetually dreamed and re-dreamed.

My dream captures the intergenerational transmission of trauma, the terror of abandonment, as well as the horror and helplessness of being the abandoning mother. In my dream, the fear of drowning, which permeates Lisa's frightening nightmares and fantasies is also a central, and alarming motif. In my dream, however, I am not frozen by the side of the pool, but frantic, desperate to find a way to escape and go-on-being, for myself and for my sons. Fighting for my life, fighting to stay alive and intact in the treatment, and fighting to help Lisa become more enlivened and less dissociated. And yet. I am still trapped in the car, feeling the great weight, the telescoping of Lisa's traumatic history (Faimberg, 2005).

Remarkably, the dream also carries messages of trauma and vulnerability from work with another patient, and another paper I had just finished writing. That paper, described in chapter three, involves a mutual survival of destructiveness, with my patient Jack, who had ridden his bike up to the George Washington Bridge, and climbed the fence to jump, only coming down at the last moment. Jack pushed me to the edge of my capacity as an analyst, and got deeply embedded in my psyche, keeping me up at night. In my dream, I am the one who goes flying off the bridge, rather than the one left behind, the one dreading that possibility.

There are even more layers complicating this dream, situating it in the socio-political moment. I presented an earlier version of this paper on a panel at IARPP in Toronto, in June 2015. The morning I was supposed to present the paper, I turned on the television in my hotel room, and heard on CNN that there had just been a terrorist attack in Tunisia, where my 26-year-old son was living, engaged in international human rights work in Tunis. Beside myself, I called him, and miraculously, he picked up the phone right away. I was flooded! with relief, hearing his voice, knowing he was safe. But it took a long time for my heart to stop racing.

Leaning on Bion's notions of dreaming and re-dreaming as *the* central analytic task and bringing my dream back to my treatment with Lisa, it captures the dizzying shock of trauma, going from laughing, warm, closeness with friends, oblivious to the dangers ahead, to being stunned—and horrified—by a sudden careening off a bridge, into deadly waters, which leads me to the next part of my story.

In our analysis, there have been periods of deep intimacy when Lisa allows herself to feel close to me, to trust me. But, even then, there's a tenuousness, a fear of losing the attachment and presence of mind, when Lisa's begged me, "Help me stay in this place, help me stay emotionally present with you." In these moments, I can feel her struggling to stay connected, to allow herself to be vulnerable, and allow me to bear and help her bear her anguish. Recently, she walked into a session, breathed deeply and said, "I'm so glad to be here." With great pride, she told me that she had bought a painting, for the first time, ever. She had never known much about art, but she saw and loved a painting in a gallery. She contacted the artist, went to her studio, and picked out a painting to buy. Lisa asks if she can show me the artist's website. It felt unusually intimate standing close together at my computer as she showed me two paintings she had chosen between. When we sat back down, in our usual positions, I told her that I liked the one she had chosen. Lisa snapped back, "I couldn't care less what you think! I bought it cause I liked it; that's what matters." I was taken aback, silenced. Destabilized by her unexpected attack, especially at that moment in such an intimate session, I was quiet, and tried to create some reflective space to find my bearings. Lisa, however, went right on talking about something else until the end of the session, unaware of the impact of her aggressive reaction.

But, neglecting to take the time to reflect on what happened between us, I got immersed in other patients' lives, and my own. I abandoned her and dissociated my hurt and shame. Lisa cancelled the next session. By the time we met, I had completely forgotten that jarring moment. In this session, I feel sleepy, bored, disengaged. Halfway through the hour, Lisa looks me in the eye and says, "What?" I ask what she is noticing. "I don't know, but something's on your mind." I say, "Something feels different today, less alive, like you're just going through the motions, not present or connected the way you've been, the way *we've* been for a while." Lisa says, "That's so weird. When I missed our last session, I thought, "I'm going to spend the next session reporting on my week, not feeling as emotionally present. I felt sad about missing our session. Maybe it felt too vulnerable or needy to admit it." Suddenly, we had both woken up from our mutual dissociation, and, in this newly open psychic space, I suddenly remember that jarring moment between us, when I shared my opinion about her choice of paintings, which we begin to explore. I say, "Hearing my opinion felt unwelcome. You felt protective of your own artistic sensibility." She nods. I continue: "But I felt surprised, hurt by your aggressive response." Lisa: "Like I slammed the door in your face." "Exactly." Tearfully, Lisa asks,

Why do I want to cry? I'm not sure why I said that. Maybe it felt too close, too threatening; it was a way of distancing you. Maybe because I respect your opinion more than anyone in the world. I needed to not be influenced by it, to trust myself with this newfound capacity to appreciate art.

When Lisa "slams the door in my face," at first I am frozen, speechless, then I dissociate the entire exchange. In the next session, I sense a deadening, but it is Lisa who notices something is on my mind, and asks me about it. It is only after Lisa asks, and I decide to share the impact she has had on me, that a mutual vulnerability becomes possible, re-opening the door to a deeper exploration of our affective experience. When Lisa says she couldn't care less what I think, I feel shamed by her and ashamed of my strong reaction, a projective identification and communication of her lifelong, un-processed shame. As I explored in chapter 2, shame travels in-sidiously across relational realms, projected and introjected from patient to analyst and back again (Levine, 2009b, 2012). Sharing my countertransference about her impact on me was powerful for Lisa, opening access to her own dissociated vulnerability and shame.

For Lisa, having a mind of her own is not a given; it must be fought for—aggressively. In her struggle to establish an authentic, self-generated identity, Lisa and I wrestle with re-experiencing and in-tegrating her traumatic past. That jarring moment between us has deep historical roots. When I intrude on her with my opinion of the painting in my attempt to join her, she is both the shamed child desperate to hold onto her fragile sense of self, and in a flash, the shaming parent who devalues, who could care less about my subjectivity. Seduction and betrayal. She does not realize the impact it has had on me, una-ware that she is identified with the aggressor, and I am the shamed, silenced child. When I "forget" this painful moment, I am the dis-sociated girl who survives by forgetting, the Old Lisa that New Lisa wants to keep buried. I am the neglectful parents, deaf and blind to the rapes endured by their daughter. Darker still, shattering the intimacy we had created, am I the seductive father/rapist who needs to be warded off to ensure her psychic survival? As I intrude on her with my opinion, I am not holding Lisa's hard-fought subjectivity in mind. Seen from this angle, when Lisa says, "I couldn't care less what you think!" she is no longer frozen or powerless; she is fighting back. It is a huge achievement that she can say, "STOP! Back off!"

It has been important to Lisa to prove to herself and to me that she is a good mother, that she will not hurt or abandon her children. In a recent session, Lisa tells me that her 20-year-old son, Jason, who has significant learning issues like Lisa, is struggling at college, overwhelmed by difficult classes, a roommate he hates, a strenuous soccer schedule. She is a fierce advocate for him, which I have supported. Lisa tells me that, the previous weekend, her husband drove up to Jason's school, met with his soccer coach and convinced him to let Jason out of his team practices, went to the registrar and helped him drop two classes, then went to the housing office to get his room changed for him. Lisa is clearly thrilled.

I meanwhile, have a powerful, judgmental reaction that I try, unsuccessfully to manage. I am thinking, "He's twenty years old. Why are they rescuing him instead of helping *him* manage the situation, supporting his independence?" I am also dimly aware of my own countertransference, that I have a son who has been struggling with the transition to adulthood, and we too wrestle with how best to support him while encouraging his independence. Clearly an area of vulnerability—and anxiety—for me. As I discussed in chapter 1, identifications with patients, overlaps in our lives and histories, can create dissociative blind spots as well as opportunities for resonance (Goldberger, 1993; Levine, 2009a). Though semi-conscious of my countertransference, I cannot seem to shift to a more empathic stance, and remain quiet. At the end of the hour, Lisa asks what I think, and in spite of myself, I wonder aloud about the way in which they are stepping in to manage the situation for Jason. Lisa looks shocked and disappointed. As soon as the words are out of my mouth, I wish I could take them back. How can I have missed that unlike her parents, Lisa is actually jumping in to rescue her drowning child? No longer the frozen mother, and proud of her protective impulse, Lisa is attempting to repair old wounds. I abandoned her, became the critical parent when she came looking for my affirmation.

In the next session, Lisa says, "I want to talk with you about something; it bothered me all week. When you asked why we're doing all this for Jason, I felt defensive. And that didn't feel right. I want to understand where you were coming from." I asked how she felt. "It took a few days to sink in. Then I got angry. I said, 'Fuck her! Yeah, 'fuck her!' I was advocating for my child, doing what I knew was in his best interest. I wasn't second-guessing myself like I usually do. I wasn't thinking, maybe she's right. I was proud of trusting myself and jumping in." Lisa, wonderfully! confronted me head on. "Fuck her! Yeah, fuck her!" Instead of feeling shamed, she found her voice, stood up to me, trusted herself in the face of my criticism. A dramatic shift.

I said, "You felt proud of how you stepped in to support Jason and wanted me to appreciate it too. Instead, you felt criticized, and you weren't afraid to tell me how angry you were." She visibly brightened. "Isn't that great? I've always been so non-confrontational."

I laughed, "Not this time."

Lisa: "Yeah, not lately. I'm like, right there."

Me: "You are! It feels so different."

Lisa: "I've never been able to do this. To try to figure out what happened when something went wrong between us. It's exciting! It feels like a collaboration."

Me: "It does, but let's not move away from your anger. You felt angry and hurt by my criticism."

Lisa: "Well, I was surprised. I was so sure we were doing the right thing for him. I expected you to support me."

Me: "I let you down."

Lisa: "Yeah, I don't want to feel like I'm going to be judged or criticized. That's not going to work for me."

Me: "I don't blame you. It feels like a big deal that you can tell me directly."

Lisa: "It's huge! Even if I felt that way in the past, I never would have brought it up so directly."

Me: "How were you able to do that?"

Lisa: "I just needed to tell you, to understand where you were coming from. But, it's hard because we know each other so well. It's not always going to go smoothly."

Me: "That's true. We're doing really deep work; we're going to affect each other. There are going to be times when we collide. But you were so honest and direct, and you trusted us to talk about it together."

Lisa: "Yeah, it feels so good. I'm going to take this and use it in other areas of my life, cause all that pushing down of my feelings gives me such anxiety. This feels much better."

Me: "You spent years pushing down your feelings, not expecting to be understood. But you had confidence in your decision to support Jason; you didn't *want* to be challenged by me. I think you also had faith that we could handle it, that our relationship could sustain the rupture and survive."

A central challenge in my work with Lisa has been to transform archaic, dissociated aggression into a form that can be enacted and processed in the transference-countertransference. The dysregulating shock of trauma is repeated, over and over, in our wounding enactments, as we each inhabit the shame-drenched roles of perpetrator, victim, and frozen bystander. But repetition is also an unconscious attempt at mastery, a sign of hope that *this time*, the reliving of trauma might turn out differently, that this time it might lead to being recognized and understood. This longing to be seen and known, to be understood from the inside out, is embedded in repetitive enactments. Lew Aron and Galit Atlas' (2015) recent work on the prospective function of enactive engagement is also relevant here. They suggest that it's not just the *working through* of enactments that's potentially generative and transformative, but the flow of enactive engagement in and of itself, as enactments are "a central means by which patient and analyst enter into each other's inner worlds and discover themselves as participants within each other's psyches" (p. 316). Enactments serve as a rehearsal, a practicing for the future, as well as a working through of the past.

In Lisa's fierce struggle to come into being, and in our mutual struggle to survive each other's ruthlessness (Winnicott, 1969) and attacks on linking (Bion, 1959), we must each struggle to recognize and own malignant "not-me" versions of ourselves (Bromberg), as we reach toward reparation and mutual recognition. And love. As Hoffman (2000) suggests,

What brings the patient into contact with the analyst's mortality, a sense that analyst and patient share a common plight, is attention to the analyst's limitations and vulnerability ... Then perhaps, our patients can integrate the need for idealization with acknowledgment that we analysts are also patients—that we are indeed, vulnerable enough, threatened enough, ... bereaved enough, traumatized enough, flawed enough, and yet also good enough, to earn the patient's empathic identification and reparative concern. (p. 845)

References

Aron, L. (1996). *A meeting of minds: Mutuality in psychoanalysis*. Hillsdale, NJ: The Analytic Press.

Aron, L. and Atlas, G. (2015). Generative enactment: Memories from the future. *Psychoanalytic Dialogues*, 25: 309–324.

Baranger, M. and Baranger, W. (2008). The analytic situation as a dynamic field. *International Journal of Psychoanalysis*, 89: 795–826.

Bass, A. (2001). It takes one to know one; or whose unconscious is it anyway? *Psychoanalytic Dialogues*, 11: 683–702.

Bion, W. (1959). Attacks on linking. *International Journal of Psychoanalysis*, 40: 308–315.

Bleger, J. (1967). Psycho-analysis of the psycho-analytic frame. *International Journal of Psychoanalysis*, 48: 511–519.

Faimberg, H. (2005). *The telescoping of generations: Listening to the narcissistic links between generations*. London: Routledge.

Ferenczi, S. (1932, 1988). *The clinical diary of Sandor Ferenczi*. Cambridge, MA: Harvard University Press.

Ferro, A. (2005). *Seeds of illness, seeds of recovery: The genesis of suffering and the role of psychoanalysis*. London: Routledge.

Ferro, A. (2006). Trauma, reverie, and the field. *Psychoanalytic Quarterly*, 75: 1045–1056.

Goldberger, M. (1993). Bright spots and blind spots.

Harris, A. (2009). You must remember this. *Psychoanalytic Dialogues*, 19: 2–21.

Hoffman, I. (2000). At death's door: Therapists and patients as agents. Psychoanalytic Dialogues, 10: 23–846.

Levinas, E. (1969). *Totality and Infinity: An essay on exteriority*. Norwell, MA: Kluwer Academic Publishers.

Levine, L. (2016). A mutual survival of destructiveness and its creative potential for agency and desire. *Psychoanalytic Dialogues*, 26: 36–49.

Levine, L. (2012). Creativity, spontaneity, impasse, and leaps of faith: Reply to commentaries. *Psychoanalytic Dialogues*, 22: 489–498.

Levine, L. (2009a). Transformative aspects of our own analysis and their resonance in our work with our patients. *Psychoanalytic Dialogues*, 19: 454–462.

Levine, L. (2009b). Impasse and resonance across multiple relational realms: Reply to commentaries. *Psychoanalytic Dialogues*, 19: 480–485.

Lyon, K., et al. (2012). Unbearable states of mind in group psychotherapy: Dissociation, mentalization, and the clinician's stance. *Group: Journal of the Eastern Group Psychotherapy Association*, 36, 4: 267–282.

Winnicott, D.W. (1969). The use of an object. *International Journal of Psycho-Analysis*, 50: 711–716.

Chapter 5

Pina Bausch: Trauma, Memory, and Creative Transformation

In the extraordinary documentary, *Pina*, Wim Wenders homage to Pina Bausch, dancers collide and fall in unexpected ways. They leap and soar, slip and fall backward or sideways, suspended momentarily in mid-air before being caught by another dancer at the last possible moment. Past and future collapse, as the powerful 3D filming transports us, the audience, right into the intensity of the present. And time falls away. It's violent, erotic, immersive.

Pina Bausch famously instructed her dancers with almost no language, encouraging them to feel their way *into* the dance, to get in touch with their deepest vulnerabilities. Central to Bausch's surreal, impassioned dance is the shock! of trauma, its violence, and haunting residue. Melancholic dancers struggle to bear trauma, to wake from the fog of dissociation, fiercely determined to break free from the ties that bind them. There's a powerful longing to connect, to embrace and be embraced. But there's trepidation, vulnerability, visible and invisible barriers to connecting. In the iconic piece, Café Mueller, dancers bump up against chairs scattered in a cafe, a couple embrace and are wrenched apart, over and over, contending with the ghosts of transgenerational trauma, which linger, reverberating and echoing, creating a sense of après-coup.

Watching Pina Bausch's dance live, especially up close, is a thrilling, evocative experience that pushes the boundaries of traditional dance performance. There's a sense that flying dancers could land in your lap, or that you could be sprayed by water splashing onto the stage when dancers leap off towering boulders. Or that you too, are a dancer on the stage, transported to another realm in your imagination. Beyond

DOI: 10.4324/9781003367475-6

being moved visually by the passionate physicality of the dance, the audience gets immersed in the affective resonance of the dancers' inner turmoil, their fervent efforts to make contact with each other, the barriers that get in the way, their struggle to mourn ineffable losses.

There is a deep embodied connection between dancers and audience, reminiscent of the essential porousness, shared vulnerability, and psychic collisions between analyst and patient. As I wrote in Chapter Four, we absorb and are penetrated by shards of our patients' trauma, and this interpenetrates with our own vulnerabilities and ungrieved losses (Harris, 2009; Levine, 2016). And as Ogden has recently written, describing the shift in psychoanalysis from an epistemological perspective of knowing and understanding to an ontological perspective of being and becoming, the goal of ontological psychoanalysis is "that of allowing the patient the experience of creatively discovering for himself, and in that state of being, becoming more fully alive" (Ogden, 2019).

In this chapter, I will focus on the intersection of trauma, creativity, and mourning. I will build on Steven Cooper's recent work on the centrality of mourning in moving from dissociation to aliveness, creativity, and the capacity to play in analysis. I resonate with Cooper's ideas about the "qualities of play catalyzed in the analytic situation to facilitate the mourning of … frustrating or unavailable objects that patients cling to through dissociated states and conscious and unconscious fantasy." I believe this mourning of unavailable or traumatizing objects entails the gradual metabolizing of shame through the analytic process, shame that fuels the repetition of old, painful patterns. Then, there is a potential opening to new enlivening object relationships, and deeper, more sustained levels of trust and intimacy.

My patient, Stefan, a talented artist, an immigrant from South America who left his homeland in early adulthood searching for a freer life, is desperately seeking a safe space, free from the intergenerational trauma that haunts him. He tells me, in our first session, that he has been in therapy twice before, but never with a woman. Women have failed to protect him, at times terrorized him. How is it that he is willing to take the risk of trusting a woman now? What is he wanting, perhaps needing, from a female analyst that he has not been able to find in his previous therapies? Stefan muses that his first therapist was too soft, his second, too harsh. "I guess I'm like Goldilocks," he says with a wry smile, "looking for a therapist who's just right."

Reflecting on Stefan's playful allusion to fairytales, and his identification with Goldilocks, in search of a therapist who is just right, I am struck by the playfulness and creativity in our dynamic right from our first session. But this was a bold challenge to me as well and perhaps held subtle power and aggression that I am not sure I, or he, was conscious of in that first meeting. I heard Stefan's message that he has a capacity and desire to play, and to play with metaphor, in his witty bid for humor, eroticism, and aliveness. I found myself compelled, drawn in, and moved by Stefan's plea for a measure of safety—inspired by his desire for creative growth and change. I felt challenged by his entreaty, by the Brombergian imperative at the heart of therapeutic action: creating a space that's safe but not too safe.

I might have felt daunted by Stefan's proposition, by the impossibility of being "just right," by the inevitability of being, at times, too hard or too soft, of our relationship becoming too hot or too cold. I knew, on some level, that I would need to be able to embrace and bear his damaging introjects which would interweave and collide with my own ungrieved losses in order for therapeutic movement and psychic change to occur. But I do not think I received a crucial aspect of this communication from him: I have already had two experiences in therapy that weren't right, that didn't help me in the ways I need help. Are you up to the task? Can I trust you? Are you going to disappoint me as well, waste my time and money? I was not yet attuned to his capacity for aggression, his identification with the aggressor in both of his parents, or to his attachment to Fairbairnian internal sabateurs and repetitive, self-destructive cycles of shame that stopped him in his tracks, that would stop us in our tracks. I did not anticipate the inevitable risks, obstacles and dangers that lay ahead in the story we were just beginning to compose together.

Goldilocks and the Three Bears can be viewed as a cautionary tale about the hazards of wandering off, the risks of exploring unknown territory, the dangers of repetition (think chairs, porridge, beds). But there are other possible interpretations. Goldilocks is a curious, risk-taking soul. The fairytale tells of a child's brave search for the right nourishment, respite and refuge from the dangers of home. However, just as Goldilocks, awoken from her slumber, flees in terror at the sudden appearance of the bear family, is Stefan also letting me know, in his identification with Goldilocks, that he can be courageous and vulnerable in exploring unknown territory, yet shut down or disappear when threatened or overwhelmed, by anger or shame, when he cannot bear to see or be seen? Was he unconsciously conveying how he holds unsymbolized terror and trauma in his body that he cannot yet express? Was he communicating the barriers to mourning and working through, which are so essential to growth and change?

Themes of presence and absence would soon become central to our work together – in the transference/countertransference, and in his old and new relationships – in his capacity for playful, creative engagement and deep intimacy, alongside his tendency to withdraw when overwhelmed by the weight of intense feelings that he is afraid he cannot bear. Stefan desperately wanted to feel more awake, less haunted, more embodied and alive. Reminiscent of Laplanche's notion of radical alterity, there is both a desire for security, a wish to be recognized and deeply understood, and a profound dread of allowing me to enter his shame-filled internal world.

Stefan tells me that he is desperately trying to free himself by leaving his tumultuous marriage after 15 years. Although his wife is an unstable, difficult person, it has not been easy to come to this decision. He feels protective of his two children, worried about his wife's controlling, critical parenting, and he agonizes over her accusations that he is abandoning his children by leaving the marriage. There are powerful intergenerational reverberations here, as his parents' stormy marriage ended with his father moving out, leaving Stefan and his older brother in the care of their psychotic mother—who then decompensated further. Stefan is scared of identifying with his father, repeating the intergenerational abandonment with his own two children. But he is terrified of identifying with his mother and her mental illness too, ashamed of his tendency to get depressed and disengage, to withdraw into himself when he gets overwhelmed. I wonder: Will I be the mama bear who scares him away? The papa bear who abandons him? How will

I inevitably—and *necessarily*—disappoint him, fall short, fail to be the therapist who is just right? Or will Stefan identify with his parents, and like Goldilocks, running away from the three bears, disappear from treatment?

In this analytic process, I imagine we will enact multiple relational configurations, and embody multiple colliding characters embedded in intergenerational trauma; perpetrator, victim, and bystander. I imagine Stefan and I will come to know many Stefans and many Laurens. We will encounter multiple ghosts from both of our pasts, and traverse numerous migratory paths together, creating a shared narrative of his traumatic history, endeavoring to work in the depressive position, and trying to imagine a more sustainable psychic future.

Deeply creative, intuitive, and self-reflective, Stefan is a talented artist who has made a career out of capturing interior life with his camera, transforming it into art. I imagine he had an early, profound longing to make inner life intelligible, to understand his mother's psychotic subjectivity, creating a container, an as-if space to manage relational trauma, a Laplanchian retranslation of his mother's enigmatic messages. Stefan expresses both guilt and sadness about his mother's limited life, and his choice to leave her behind when he came to the U.S. to create a life of his own, a crucial step in separating from her, physically and psychologically. Although his mother died years ago, he speaks wistfully about a fantasy that he could bring her here to New York, to see his life, meet his children.

But this mother, about whom he imagines seeing his life and appreciating all that he has created, is not the mother who terrified him in her manic states, or the mother who retreated into depression and self-absorption. It is the mother he glimpsed occasionally; the fantasied mother he still longs for, waits for, a mother who will recognize him, hold him, be present and enlivening. And the life he wishes she could witness does not include the shame he often feels about his struggle to stay motivated and engaged, to move forward in his work and relationships.

Stefan tells me he is afraid he has lost himself, lost his voice, over the course of his difficult marriage. I wonder how he managed to have a voice at all, and how he lost it; how he learned as a little boy to protect himself, an adaptive defense of withdrawing, of hiding to protect himself from his mother's unpredictable and frightening behavior. His descriptions of encountering his mother in the hallway of their apartment, staring at him with hollow eyes, as if seeing right through him, are haunting, eerie, evocative of a Pina Bauschian scene with one dancer desperately trying to connect with another who is cut off, dissociated, staring off into space, in her own world. I see the frightened little boy in front of me; hear his pleas for connection, and his fear of intimacy, as the moments of connection are fragile and unpredictable.

This brings to mind Seligman's (2016) ideas about the intricate dance of mother-infant interaction and how a mother's attuned response to her infant's spontaneous gesture essentially transforms the movement over time and space to create intersubjective communication, temporality, and vitality, giving the baby "compelling evidence of her effect on the world" (p. 225). Like Julia in Chapter Two, Stefan had a strong desire to "embody" himself more, to feel more enlivened and agentic. According to Seligman, when a mother is not responsive to an infant's gestures, or only intermittently responsive, like Stefan's mother, there is no sense of time moving forward, only "the stasis of a present which never gives way to an emergent future." How could Stefan and I create a consistent sense of time moving forward, a sense of his own agency and creative potential in the face of challenging obstacles?

Stefan tells me that his wife has been accusing him of emotionally abandoning her and their children, as she accused him throughout their marriage, complaining for years about his "checking out," about his tendency to dissociate. This was a central issue in their couples therapy he tells me. With great anguish, he says, looking out the window of my office, "I hate that word, 'dissociate.'"

I am not sure what happened at that moment, but I could feel, in his hatred of the word dissociate, the self-loathing he felt in being accused of being someone who checks out, a mother who becomes depressed or manic, a father who disappears. And yet, I imagined the little boy who needed desperately to ward off his mother's psychotic episodes in order to protect his own sanity. I could feel both his self-protective need to check out, his need to rely on his imaginative inner life, and his profound longing to be seen and recognized. I took a risk, as this was a man I was just beginning to get to know. Yet, I felt connected to Stefan, and I understood, on a visceral level, his need for self-preservation.

When Stefan said despondently to me, "I hate that word, dissociate," I responded, "Stefan, I think dissociation saved your life. I think it served a crucial self-protective function for you." He looked at me with a sense of shock, with eyes wide open, and began to weep. And then sob. We sat quietly together. "No one's ever said that to me before," he spoke through his tears. "I always felt like I was so fucked up for 'checking out'. And my ex used it as a weapon against me, telling me I was a bad husband and father because I dissociated so much." In the next session, he told me what a revelation—and profound relief, that was to hear:

It made me feel normal for the first time. I never considered that my checking out might have been how I protected myself as a child, from the fear of my mother, and the anger at my father for leaving me behind with my mother.

These sessions felt deeply moving and intimate. But my reframing of dissociation, though revelatory and affirming to Stefan, was just the beginning, the first step of a complex, nonlinear, transference/countertransference journey of both understanding the function of dissociation, and moving from dissociation toward what Bromberg calls, standing in the spaces, an ability to be more present, to hold multiple, conflicting self-states, and share those shameful, self-loathing parts of himself with me.

Along these lines, Stefan shares with me months later that sometimes he does not want to come to sessions, that he worries about being judged by me. "Tell me," I responded. He says:

This feels hard to say, to tell you, but even though I feel affirmed by you— your faith in me feels so important, I'm also aware of editing out parts of myself that don't fit with the sensitive man I feel reflected back to me. I think I've felt afraid of bringing in those parts of myself, not knowing how you'll respond, if you'll still care about me, if you'll still see me as a good person, a good man. I worry that it will taint the image you have of me.

I'm struck by the poignancy of Stefan's admission, of his courage in this moment, challenging both of us to go further and deeper, allowing him to begin to bring in more shameful, hidden parts of himself. This was also important supervision to me, piercing a degree of idealization I had held of him, enabling me to see ways in which I had, in some ways minimized his more aggressive and self-destructive parts. It opened a door to seeing him with more complexity, recognizing the insidious impact of early relational trauma, and potentially allowing him to feel more fully seen and known by me.

I said: "Stefan, I'm glad you could share that with me, that it's felt hard to share parts of yourself with me, that you're afraid you'll lose my caring and faith in you. How were you able to tell me now?" Stefan responded:

It just felt important. I want to get to a better place, to work through the barriers that get in the way of moving forward with my life, to feel more awake and present. And I know I can't do that by hiding from you, by hiding shameful parts of myself.

"That's true," I said. "But I'm curious about my role in reflecting back affirmation and faith in you, which I do feel, but maybe not leaving enough space for aspects of you that conflict with the sensitive, creative soul, the aggressive and self-destructive parts."

Then Stefan began to share, for the first time, how he drinks and smokes weed every night, that he can spend endless hours on the internet, lose himself, dissociate from the angst of his impending divorce, his wife's angry texts about what a bad husband and father he's been, and his desire to procrastinate in doing his taxes, or his billing for his business, or other adult obligations he wishes to avoid. Recently, he told me he had had a physical where his doctor told him his drinking was affecting his health, and that he needed to start taking better care of himself. He said it was a wake-up call, that he wants to try to be healthier.

I began to pay more attention to Stefan's rage and identification with his mother, and her capacity for psychic violence, in his anger at his soon to be ex-wife. He responded to her toxic texts with his own hefty hate and aggression, and there was ferocity in their texting attacks and counter-attacks. Her cruelty could be dysregulating, send him into shameful, self-deprecating retreats. I worked with him to separate from her, to see her poisonous texts as an effort to get under his skin, to keep him engaged with her, as she was both saddened and enraged by his leaving her. But we also talked about his own aggression and destructiveness, not just as a reaction to his wife, but in its own right. We talked about how he struggles to stay connected to his adolescent children and that he can go days or weeks without reaching out to them, if they don't reach out to him, especially when he's busy traveling for work, and how harmful that is for his kids. He was open in these conversations, saying he wants to feel more consistently present and connected to his children, but clearly old dissociative and avoidant patterns are difficult to break.

Though it was clear to me early on in the affection with which he talked about them, Stefan seemed to minimize his vital importance to his children. I encouraged him to reach out more regularly to them, emphasized that it mattered, even when they were being unresponsive teenagers. Although he felt he had not been consistently emotionally present with his children during his marriage, a deep source of shame for him, it was apparent to me that his children loved him deeply, and that he was a loving, more flexible, less controlling parent. It moved him to realize how deeply attached his kids were to him, and as he called and texted more often, he felt closer to them, and they, in turn, were more responsive to him. Moving out of shame and self-loathing toward self-compassion has been a central, nonlinear, and ongoing challenge in the therapy, as shame is about not wanting to be seen in one's entirety, in one's messiness and complexity.

After he separated from his wife, Stefan rented an apartment near his children so he could more easily spend time with them. He described the apartment to me with excitement: "It was a nondescript building in a nondescript neighborhood," Stefan said, "but when I walked into the apartment, what I saw was a big picture window overlooking the Hudson River. It felt like a window onto another world." We sat together quietly as I took this in. I imagined this space, as he painted it for me in his vivid descriptions. I associated to the film, Pina, as Wim Wenders' 3D window into the essence of Pina Bausch's dance. I commented on Stefan's wish to be transported into another world, beyond the trauma, both past and present. "A refuge," I said, and he replied, "Yes, absolutely."

I wondered how he learned to do that as a child, find ways of being transported into other worlds, away from the chaos at home. Then I had an association to the novel, *Exit West*, by the Pakistani writer, Mohsin Hamid, a story about migration across space, time, and culture, a story in which two desperate refugees fall in love and are magically transported through portals to new worlds, where they risk their lives in the hope of finding safety and security. But their respite is temporary, as each new city brings harsh political realities for refugees, who bring their cultural and relational trauma with them, which weighs on them as the past gets enacted in the present.

Stefan has also fallen in love, and he and his partner, also an artist, have had many adventures and magical times together, even as they have bumped up against obstacles working to integrate their individual lives. Stefan tells me how important it feels to be creating a new home, for himself, his partner, and his children. He tells me how preoccupied he has been, like Goldilocks, about finding and building a home that's just right. He stays up late into the night looking at furniture and materials and lighting online. He invites his kids to help with projects like building shelves, choosing colors and painting the walls of their rooms, designing menus and cooking together. They identify with Stefan's creativity and artistic aesthetic, join him in this home-building. These are close family moments. From our first conversations, I have been moved by Stefan's artistic sensibility, and the joy he gets from creating art. Stefan approaches every creative endeavor with great care, and an artistic eye: cooking, photography, creating a home.

I have been struck too, by his access to profound pain. Our sessions are often moving and intimate, with a mutual sense of creativity and flow, a sense of being in time together, as Stefan has the capacity to drop into the past, getting in touch with deep vulnerability and anguish. But partly because of his job which requires international travel, and because of his difficulty staying connected to me and to our analytic process, this mutual sense of flow does not last. It feels both deep and ephemeral. Working through childhood trauma is enormously challenging.

A part of Stefan remains frozen, traumatized by a bipolar mother and an abandoning father. Although he is desperate to leave his past behind, to heal from his early trauma and abandonment, his body keeps him trapped in the past, with wordless emotions and feelings and nameless dread. Like Pina Baush's dancers, struggling to bear trauma, to wake from the fog of dissociation, to break free from the ties that bind them. While there is a powerful longing to connect, to embrace and be embraced, there's trepidation, vulnerability, visible and invisible barriers to connecting.

While Stefan can be strikingly open and vulnerable, he can suddenly disengage, move in and out of touch, appearing and disappearing, cancelling sessions and taking breaks from therapy. Sometimes the cancellations are due to work commitments requiring travel; other times out of anger and frustration that therapy, *that I,* cannot seem to help him move forward and create change in his life. And sometimes he just disappears, and I cannot find him, a projective identification of his experience of maternal and paternal abandonment. Then I feel the pain of his disappearing, of his sudden departures without warning, the impossibility of convincing him to stay and work through the impasse, through the mourning, to get to a less dissociated, more connected place.

At these times when he withdraws from me, he often retreats more generally from relationships and work responsibilities accompanied by a loss of play and creativity in his own inner world. Shutting down into a shame-filled place where he feels utterly alone, Stefan loses touch with any sense of connection, motivation, or agency. He finds it difficult to consistently take action to move forward in his life, with work, with his divorce. He struggles to do the financial and accounting work that divorce entails, caught in cycles of procrastination, self-blame, and shame.

We have frequently talked about his retreating into a little boy self-state of wishing a parent would take care of him, feeling alone, abandoned, and humiliated, wishing I would be the mother he never had, but always wished for, is still wishing for. I am aware of both the desire, the pull to rescue him from the abyss of despair, and the impossibility of this, of being the mother who can enliven and motivate him. This longing to be taken care of—rescued – causes him deep shame and brings him in touch with both the poignant wish and the impossibility of turning back time.

Although we have discussed both strategies to stay engaged and connected with his work and other obligations and delving into the past to understand the dynamic roots of these patterns, Stefan struggles to consistently move away from old and deeply frustrating patterns of presence and absence, immobilization and stuckness. He gets angry at me for not helping him break this old, upsetting dynamic. He has said some version of the following more than once:

> Yeah, yeah, I know, I wish you could be the loving mom, the attentive mother I never had, that you could help me feel less alone with my pain, that you could keep me from spiraling into the rabbit hole of despair, to stay focused and motivated, but so what? That isn't helping me change this shitty dynamic that makes me feel like such a mess, such a failure. Long pause. I feel so ashamed.

Furious at himself and at me, Stefan then distances himself from me, cancels sessions, and does not return my calls or texts, saying he wants to take a break from therapy.

I can see his identification with both parents in his periodic disappearing, in his withdrawal. Acutely sensitive to feeling abandoned, his impulse is to abandon the other, identify with the abandoner, leaving his partner, child, or me feeling hurt, shocked, angry. I knew, on some level, that we needed to enact these dynamics in the transference/countertransference if we were to experience and process the chaos and abandonment he was subjected to as a child. But I felt as if every time we got closer to processing these painful feelings, Stefan disappeared. He and I both felt frustrated by his stuckness, his feeling stuck in time, unable to move his life forward in real time, and our inability to go deeper, to make use of our analytic understanding by Stefan's withdrawing every time he was making progress.

But I also tried to hold in mind, and help Stefan hold in mind, the nonlinearity of growth and change, that embedded in repetition, there are aspects of hope, as well as shame (Harris, 2009).

Steven Cooper (2022) writes about the challenge of helping patients understand the cost of these toxic attachments in real time, as part of a mourning process. He writes that in play, the analyst is "occupying territory between the patient's different self-states associated with these attachments that are often not on speaking terms with one another. The analyst has to get inside these places of discontinuity, dissociated states and fixed attachment." Cooper writes "about *the play of mourning*," that forms of play can help patients acknowledge the need to gain distance from and mourn unavailable or frustrating others.

Stefan's mother was hospitalized several times in his early life. During those hospitalizations, his grandparents brought him back to their home and wrote letters to his father about how Stefan was doing, letters which Stefan recently found. I asked if he wanted to bring them in, and he spread them out like a fan on the floor between us in dated order, and translated them into English, tearfully. It was one of those poignant moments when he dropped back in time as he talked about memories of his mother's depressions and hospitalizations, and the comfort of his grandparents' care. I had embodied associations to my days of doing play therapy, sitting on the floor playing with a young child patient, acting out their family story. I had a powerful sense of how Stefan must have felt with his depressed mother, his dread of her deadness, his desperate need/desire to stay enlivened himself. Stefan's psychic retreats can make me feel helpless and alone, and I'm aware of a pull "to create presence in the space left by absence" (Gerson, 2009).

For someone who uses his camera for a living and for his art, Stefan had a difficult time shifting to zoom during the pandemic, and almost immediately decided to take a break until we could resume in person. While I tried to explore experimenting with working virtually or by phone, Stefan was adamant. He said he could not imagine doing deep work and connecting across a screen. Six months later, still in the midst of the pandelic, he reached out, willing to give it a try, which we did for four months, until he wanted to suspend sessions yet again. I am still waiting, hoping to hear from Stefan, hoping to continue our compelling work on mourning, creativity, and aliveness.

The film, *Pina*, an elegy to Pina Bausch, holds multiple layers of trauma and creativity, trauma interrupting/disrupting creativity, and then creativity reimagined, re-enlivened, and co-created as transitional object. Reminiscent of Ogden's (2000) notion of mourning as:

A demand to create something … a memory, a dream, a story, a poem, that begins to meet, to be equal to, the full complexity of our relationship to what has been lost. Paradoxically, in this process, we are enlivened by the experience of loss and death, even when what is given up or taken from us is an aspect of ourselves. (p. 65)

While writing this chapter, I had a dream, a time traveling dream of my own. In the dream, I was looking for a quiet place to read. I felt a distinct sense that it was getting late, that I was *running out of time.* Suddenly, I found myself in my childhood apartment, and I walked into my parents' old bedroom. My mother, who died nine years ago, before *her* time, was lying on her bed reading, very much alive. I had no sense of this being strange, of her having died, as I was *back in time with her.* "Can I read here with you, mom?" I asked. "Sure," she responded, and patted the space next to her on the bed. Just then, I noticed a naked baby laying on the bed, a beautiful baby girl, and I leaned over to smell her baby smell, to feel her baby skin on my skin.

This dream holds a dizzying array of self-states across time, a lifetime, a reawakening and a rebirth. It holds aspects of memory and desire, attachment and mourning, ghosts of mothers, and babies. I am aware of myself as reader and writer, embodying my adult, creative self, as mother and baby, mother to Stefan, to his adult and younger selves. There is a longing for my mother, for snuggling and bedtime stories, longing for a safe refuge. And Stefan's longing for his mother, and connection to his children, to his maternal/paternal self-states. There is wistfulness about the passage of time, aging, and mortality. Nostalgia as a mother, for those early days when my now grown sons were babies, sensory memories of soft baby skin and delicious baby smells. There are multiple dimensions of time: running out of time, being back in time, the fantasy of stopping time—of staying right here, right now, forever.

My dream undoes time, undoes death, takes place in the liminal space of mortality, in the realm of the melancholic. It captures aspects of my work with Stefan, ways in which he moves toward and away from me, toward and away from his own grief and trauma, from dissociation to aliveness and creativity and back again. It conjures questions raised in chapter two about the ways in which patients' access to their imagination, dreams, and other unconscious realms interweaves with the analyst's variable and shifting receptivity to her own imagination and creativity.

My dream evokes the nonlinearity of time in analysis, a Laplanchian re-transcribing of traumatic experience. Both Stefan's and my fantasies of being reunited with a loving mom, my re-enlivened mother's making space for me next to her on the bed, a wish to be that loving, attuned mother/analyst for Stefan, the need for both of us to mourn that fantasy. And the desire and longing for intimacy and connection, so hard to sustain.

I saw the documentary, *Pina*, the first time, with *my mother,* who had been a dancer in her younger days. When it was over, we were both so blown away by the embodied intensity and traumatic urgency of the film that we could not stand up right away. We had to catch our breaths. As if we ourselves had been dancing the duets in the film.

Every artist is a constellation of influences, a messy composite of other people and past experiences. In dance, that entanglement is especially intimate, deeply rooted in the body. Whose work is it? Where does the choreographer end and the dancer begin? We *are* aspects of the people we have known, even those who are no longer here. They too are present in the dance.

Velleda Ceccoli (2012) writes:

> Pina Bausch wasn't just interested in how people move, but rather, what moves *them* ... Dance emerges as the very basis of a different language, the language of human experience accessing emotions directly—then she goes further, into the emotional resonance of others. Dance thus becomes the language of trauma re-worked and extended through our common bond – our humanity. Her dance becomes the means of accessing narratives that escape the preciseness of language, yet demand to be understood, processed, and finally spoken.

Ceccoli continues,

> Bausch created a direct link to our emotions speaking to us through multiple narratives of movement, music, theater and performance. Her work addresses our first language, the language of affect, a language that needs no translation. The bodies of her dancers become its creator, carrier, choreographer and narrator."

In her dreamlike dance-theater, Pina Bausch takes a fearless look at human relationships, and takes the full range of human emotions as her starting point.

Pina was created in the wake of tragedy and shocking loss. It was originally a joint project, a thrilling collaboration between Wim Wenders and Pina Bausch. But Bausch died suddenly and unexpectedly in the process of making the film. Devastated, Wenders walked away from the project. But the dancers in her company, Tanztheater Wuppertal, pleaded with him to come back, to not abandon the film. After many months, Wenders decided that the only way he could make the film was to *re*-make it, to create a new version, no longer *with Pina* but *for* her—an elegy to *Pina*. And he felt he needed to make it in 3D, to capture the power and full-bodied aliveness of Bausch's immersive choreography. Pina is above all, an act of preservation, a memorial that is also a defiance of mortality—completely alive in every dimension. Transforming trauma into art.

Pina Bausch's work, like psychoanalysis, like my work with Stefan, involves play and improvisation, reckoning with attachment and trauma, love and loss. Living passionately in the present requires the mourning of trauma in the service of growth and change, struggling to work, and help our patients work, in the depressive position (Cooper, 2016a and b). It requires reckoning with the bittersweet, and inevitable incompleteness of our work, accepting our own limitations and the inexorableness of mortality.

References

Ceccoli, V. (2012). Feeling Pina: How the choreographer moved people. http://psychologytomorrowmagazine.com/feeling-pina-how-the-choreographer-moved-people, November 5, 2012.

Cooper, S. (2016a). Mourning, regeneration, and the psychic future: A discussion of Levine's "A mutual survival of destructiveness and its creative potential for agency and desire". *Psychoanalytic Dialogues*, 26: 56–62.

Cooper, S. (2016b). *The Melancholic Errand of Psychoanalysis: Exploring the Analyst's Relationship to the Depressive Position*. London: Routledge.

Cooper, S. H. (2022). The limits of intimacy and the intimacy of limit: Play and its relation to the bad object. *Journal of the American Psychoanalytic Association*, 70, 241–261.

Gerson, S. (2009). When the third is dead: Memory, mourning, and witnessing in the aftermath of the Holocaust. In Relational Psychoanalysis. *Expansion of theory*, Vol. 4, 347–366.

Harris, A. (2009). You must remember this. *Psychoanalytic Dialogues*, 19: 2–21.

Levine (2016). Mutual vulnerability: Intimacy, psychic collisions, and the shards of trauma. *Psychoanalytic Dialogues*, 26: 571–579.

Ogden, T. (2000). Borges and the art of mourning. *Psychoanalytic Dialogues*, 10, 65–88.

Ogden, T. (2019). Ontological Psychoanalysis or 'What Do You Want to Be When You Grow Up?'. *The Psychoanalytic Quarterly*, 88: 4, 661–684.

Seligman, S. (2016). Disorders of temporality and the subjective experience of time: Unresponsive objects and the vacuity of the future. *Psychoanalytic Dialogues*, 26: 110–128.

Chapter 6

Finding Creative Means of Staying Enlivened when Locked in an Endless Present: Deconstructing the Film *Room*

In the heart-wrenching film, *Room*, an adolescent girl, ironically named Joy, is abducted, imprisoned, and impregnated by her captor. When the film opens, her son, Jack is five years old, and Joy has been held captive for seven long years, with no hope of escape. Though Jack is the product of rape, he gives Joy something *essential* to live for. She's fiercely protective, and determined to create an imaginative, even joyful world for her son within the confines of Room. This desperate imperative, Winnicott's *primary maternal preoccupation* as a means of survival, enables Joy to channel the chaos of her ongoing trauma and despair into a creative, life-sustaining endeavor. However, Winnicott theorized primary maternal preoccupation as a temporary period following the birth of an infant ("a temporary illness from which the mother spontaneously recovers"). What happens when maternal preoccupation doesn't feel temporary, or when it's freighted with the urgency of survival? I will come back to this point about primary maternal preoccupation as both essential—life-saving—for Joy and soaked with trauma.

For Jack, Room is the whole world, all he has ever known, and to some extent, he seems content and full of wonder, living there with Ma. But Joy has a doubled consciousness. She has to manage the nearly impossible task of creating a safe, growth-enhancing home for her son in Room, while reckoning with her own ongoing anguish, knowing the real world is going-on-being in her absence—that time is moving forward, Jack is growing taller, older, marking time, even as they're trapped in an interminable present.

DOI: 10.4324/9781003367475-7

In this chapter, I will explore the human capacity for resilience in the face of unspeakable trauma, the challenge of finding creative means of staying enlivened, when locked in an endless present. I will draw on Viktor Frankl's philosophical writing on the crucial importance of finding meaning, even under the harshest conditions. Frankl (1959), psychiatrist, philosopher, and Holocaust survivor built on Nietzsche's idea that "he who has a Why to live for can bear almost any How." Frankl believed that although we cannot avoid suffering, we can choose how we cope with it—that finding meaning even under the most brutal circumstances can be life-sustaining. Frankl's work has echoes of Sartrean existentialism. As Sartre suggested, even war, imprisonment, or the prospect of imminent death cannot take away our existential freedom, that we must "remain passionately, furiously engaged with life, at all costs (Bakewell, 2016)."

I will also draw on Bryan Stevenson's (2014) remarkable book, *Just Mercy*, which traces the insidious legacy of slavery, racial violence and trauma embedded in American history and their impact on the vast racial inequities of mass incarceration. Stevenson, a civil rights attorney, founded and directs the Equal Justice Initiative, whose lawyers represent indigent men, women and children, many innocent, or unjustly accused, trapped in the furthest reaches of our prison system, in solitary confinement or death row, with little hope of a future. Stevenson's reach, in *Just Mercy*, is broad and deep; historical, political, and deeply personal. He tells stories of trauma, survival, and resilience, emphasizing the crucial importance of witnessing and storytelling in restoring human dignity.

I am going to read the film *Room* from multiple, overlapping perspectives in regard to trauma. The film itself is told from several perspectives, as Jack's reflections are interspersed throughout the film. In the opening scene, we see Joy and Jack waking up in a shared bed in a small room, and we hear Jack's voiceover, telling us a story, his birth story actually, or at least the all too disturbing fairy tale his Ma has told him. It is a dark fairy tale, to be sure, and Jack is the hero at the center, who saves his Ma, as he does in the film, again and again. It begins, as most fairytales do, with Once Upon a Time.

Jack tells us that once upon a time, before he was born, his Ma *cried and cried*, and watched TV all day long, till she became a zombie. But then he *zoomed* down from Heaven into Room.

Whooooosh!! He was kicking Ma from inside and then he shot out onto Rug with his eyes *wide open*, and Ma said, *"Hello, Jack!"*

There is *so* much; in fact, a "too-muchness" captured in Jack's heartbreaking introductory monologue. Joy has told Jack a version of his birth story that has much truth – and *so much trauma*. Jack is, right from the beginning, interpellated into the role of superhero and savior of his traumatized mother. Joy has consciously excised her captor and rapist, Jack's biological father, from the story. This birth story is the first sign of Laplanchian enigmatic traumatic messages communicated from mother to son, the paradox of the loving, maternal, playful mom and the traumatized mom, the many ways in which Joy isn't containing the trauma, but translating and transmitting it to Jack through what Laplanche calls, intromission, a violent and "utterly untranslatable" form of trauma, that "thwarts the subject's freedom to develop his own subjectivity" (Scarfone, 2017, p. 41). As Scarfone poetically describes:

> Not all traumas are the same. There are structuring traumas, on the side of weaving living systems, and traumas that tear apart, disorganize, paralyze, and disorient ... Implantation is of the structuring kind, while intromission belongs to the second, deleterious form of seduction.
>
> (Laplanche, 1990, p. 26)

This question about the degree to which Jack is both protected and traumatized by Joy's severe, ongoing trauma is an open question, one which the film doesn't take up, per se, but which I will explore in this chapter.

In addition to the manifest narrative, we can imagine Room as the room of the consulting room, in terms of the complexity of bearing witness when treating massive trauma; the challenge of creating a container, an as-if space to manage the reliving and processing of trauma, as both analyst and patient can often feel trapped in an endless present. Sometimes our Rooms can feel like sanctuaries. And sometimes they can feel like prisons. This puts a tremendous demand on the analyst, as I have written in several chapters, as analysts absorb and are penetrated by shards of our patients' trauma, which bump up against and interpenetrate with our traumatic histories.

However, unlike Joy, for whom Winnicott's primary maternal preoccupation served a crucial survival function, in the consulting room, we say "we have to stop now," a reminder that our preoccupation with our patients, our witnessing and deep involvement with their needs and traumas, has boundaries, and is not unending in the same way. The frame, at least to some extent, keeps us from the interminable present with which Joy contends in her maternal preoccupation.

Room can be read as a psychoanalytic text about a woman trapped in the room of her own mind, imprisoned in her traumatic past. We can understand the film as flashbacks, nightmares, ways in which trauma lives on in us as frozen repetition, how it can be denied, dissociated, unwitnessed, and unmourned. Time collapses in the face of trauma, as past and future become entangled, lose their meaning, fall away (Harris and Bartlett, 2016; Levine, 2018). Like Joy, we can feel caught in an *unending present* with our most challenging, traumatized patients.

The different *characters* in the film can be read as dissociated parts of Joy, self-states that get enacted in the treatment of trauma, as analyst and patient variously take on the roles of perpetrator, victim, bystander or witness. But there are other self-states here too that need to be recognized and honored; an overwhelming love, *mother love*, an attuned, creative mother-love, resilient parts of Joy that she is able to mobilize because of Jack's existence and their profound attachment, to help manage the nightmare of her imprisonment.

Speaking of mother love, it is striking that, although Jack is five years old, Joy has continued to breastfeed him throughout their captivity in Room. We can understand this as Joy's effort to hold onto the skin-to-skin contact and bodily intimacy, Anzieu's skin ego, as well as the enlivening, eroticized experience of breastfeeding, creating a liminal, visceral space of love and nurturance in the midst of all the horror. We might also imagine a wish to stop time, to hold onto a nurturing, maternal self-state, the fantasy that she can protect and sustain Jack, in part to ward off the hate and destructiveness she feels toward her captor. Perhaps it's also a way of "nursing" her own wounds, trying to fill her own emptiness and hopelessness, an effort at self-care. To what extent is Joy using Jack to fulfill her own desperate needs, in order to survive the massive trauma she is undergoing?

The film can also be understood as a mother's fierce attempt to protect her child from the intergenerational transmission of trauma (Salberg and Grand, 2017). In the small room in which they are trapped, Joy creates a stimulating, loving home for Jack, with homework, daily exercise, creative play, and other maternal and self-care. She has created rituals, like hiding Jack in the closet before their captor, Nick, unlocks the door and enters Room each night, violating their private world. She has made the closet into a cozy little nest, reading Jack a bedtime story, and putting a headset on him, so he does not witness her degrading nightly violations. Joy submits noiselessly to being raped, to protect Jack from Nick's violence and rage.

Jack does not know, consciously at least, that their captor is his biological father, and Joy is determined that he not find out, that she keep the toxicity of his (and her) legacy a secret. She tries to rewrite the story, creating a fictionalized fairy tale for Jack, to help him deal with his terror of her captor, whom she names *Old Nick,* giving him a fairy tale "pretend" designation, as if he were just a make believe bad guy, to mitigate the traumatic impact on Jack. But, as we all know, fairy tales can be right on the edge of terrifying. Though Joy creates an as-if world of make-believe for Jack, her devastation and despair leak through, just as Jack can hear through the slats of the closet what Old Nick does to his Ma every night. And, of course the ritual of putting Jack in a closet to protect him has a doubled meaning, as it can also be likened to Joy's dissociation, a closeting, or walling off of her own affective experience to protect herself, as well as Jack, from her nightly trauma.

Joy wants to protect Jack at all costs from the trauma she has endured and continues to endure. She cannot bear to face the idea that Jack is being traumatized by the hell she is undergoing. As I wrote in the beginning, "this desperate imperative, Winnicott's primary maternal preoccupation as a means of survival, enables her to channel the chaos of her ongoing trauma and despair into a life-sustaining endeavor."

However, Joy continually struggles to manage her anguish, rage, and depression. It is only when she is able to perceive the impact her frustration and anger have on Jack that she manages to contain her aggressive impulses, and reach out to Jack lovingly, to repair the damage. Her awareness that there is a world out there that she is missing, a family, a life outside Room, at times breaks through her dissociation, and then she shuts down completely, for hours at a time. For those hours, it is as if she is experiencing a kind of psychic death, or what Laub (2017a) calls "a profound state of inner lonesomeness … objectlessness, with an absence of communicable thought." And what about Jack? When Ma succumbs to this "state of inner lonesomeness," she disappears psychically; she becomes Andre Green's "dead mother." The container cracks, and Joy cannot protect Jack from the transmission of trauma. Jack has learned by age five, by the time we meet him, that when Ma is in this dissociated objectless state, he must fend for himself. He must rely on his deeply creative imagination to keep himself company—and try to ward off witnessing his Ma in such a tortured, vulnerable state.

The film portrays Jack as resilient and adaptive, which he surely is, but it does not explore the damage we can surmise he may have internalized from his mother's trauma, depression and deadness, and his witnessing of her nightly rapes. As Salberg (2015) indicates. "The child shapes himself to fit a parent's wound of history, be it war, rape, slavery, death" (p. 37). Salberg suggests that in order to attach to a traumatized parent, the child "will need to enter and become enmeshed in the trauma scene … so that the parent's trauma story enters the child's cellular makeup before there are words, and thus a narrative can be told" (p. 37).

When the film begins, it is Jack's fifth birthday. So we, the audience, are not privy to Joy's abduction or her early years in captivity. We are spared that trauma. By the time we are introduced to Room, Joy is no longer in solitary confinement; she already has a point of reference, a connection to the world of the social—and a funny, stimulating, creative companion. She has a kind of witness in five year-old Jack. But, it is a *limited, complicated, compromised* kind of witnessing. And crucially, Jack cannot serve as witness to Joy because his very existence holds and mirrors the trauma itself.

Further, Jack cannot bear witness to the overwhelming torment Joy is continuing to experience, as Joy tries her best to *hide* it from him. While Joy has Jack for company, and focuses all her energy on taking care of him, on another level, she is still utterly alone, imprisoned in her traumatic experience, as her inner torment is still private, compartmentalized, unspeakable. And she is literally trapped, incarcerated by her captor.

One of the readings that has been instrumental in my reading of the film is Bryan Stevenson's (2014) book, *Just Mercy*, about the horrors and racial inequities of our criminal justice system. Stevenson describes the intergenerational transmission of trauma in many incarcerated individuals' histories, trauma that has been ignored in harsh, inequitable sentencing. On the most intimate level, Stevenson also writes about the importance of serving as a witness, listening to his clients' testimony, to horrendous stories of abuse and neglect, and offering a depth of humanity in the context of a dehumanizing prison system.

Stevenson tells the story of his first visit to a federal penitentiary, back when he was a legal intern, inexperienced and terrified to visit a man who had been in solitary confinement for many years. He then describes his shock, coming face to face with just another frightened human being, an African American man like himself, exactly the same age, inordinately grateful for the opportunity for human contact. Stevenson was there to tell the man that his execution had been stayed for at least the next year. The man was overjoyed. The visit was only supposed to last an hour, but they talked for three—about music, family, life outside. What Stevenson had been afraid of in entering this prison was the man's Otherness. But what ensued was a profound moment of meeting, a powerful shift from objectification to mutual recognition. When Stevenson was forced by the guards to leave, the man, handcuffed and shackled, stood up, head held high, and started to sing a gospel song, a song of resistance, with renewed dignity, having had the experience of witnessing—of being heard, respected, and humanized.

But what happens after years of imprisonment, if one's lucky enough to be released, or to escape? Once Joy and Jack manage to escape from Room, a new phase of trauma takes hold for Joy. In yet another profound way in which Jack saves Joy from descending into despair, Jack is the one who escapes and saves them from captivity. It's a terrifying, heart-stopping flight into freedom. Joy comes up with a plan to pretend that Jack has died from an untreated illness, wraps Jack in a rug, and convinces Old Nick to take his body to bury him. Ma directs Jack on exactly how to unroll from the rug, and jump out from the back of Old Nick's pickup truck, once they are in a neighborhood with people around. Though Old Nick tries to stop Jack from escaping, Jack manages to get away, and is rescued by a neighbor, who calls the police, who then reunite Jack and his Ma. It is an overwhelming, tearful reunion, and watching this scene of reunification as the mother of two sons, it's almost unbearable. Such relief from the horror of seven years of captivity and trauma, immeasurable relief that Jack and his Ma are reunited.

And yet. Joy's immense relief and joy in being free and back with Jack and later, with her family dissipates within days, replaced by a gaping wound, the horror of what has happened. While trapped in Room, Jack served a containing and meaning-making function for her. But now, Joy is flooded by what Gerson (2009) calls "the enduring presence of an absence," the unbearable reality of what she has lost, what has been taken from her. She cannot turn back time, or erase the past. Instead, she has to wrestle with *feeling* erased.

Similarly, Laub (2017b) describes what happened to many Holocaust survivors after the war, including his own mother, who was intrepid and resilient beyond imagination during the war, then fell apart afterward. Laub writes that, like Joy, in the concentration camp, his mother's "primary and most coveted wish was to ferociously protect her only child from experiencing the harsh reality they all lived in" (p. 28). She "could not share her terror or her worries … She had to appear steadfast and self-assured so as to keep *his* spirits up … even when she felt the ground under her feet giving way" (p. 24). But, after the war, after they got *through* the horror, his mother never recovered, and sadly experienced a life of pain and *unending mourning*.

In the seven years Joy has been missing, her family has fallen apart. Her parents have separated, her mother has found a new partner, and her father cannot bear to face the trauma of what has happened to his only child. He cannot even look at Jack, as he is both horrified and disgusted by the product of his daughter's rape. Joy and Jack are Othered by her father, repudiated, tainted. Joy angrily, and desperately, asks her father to look at Jack. He cannot or will not. This is unspeakably shaming and objectifying of Jack, as well as Joy—seeing him only as the embodiment of his daughter's trauma, a not infrequent response from family and community to sexual violence. Jack is everything to Joy, her most primary attachment and only connection to a future, *quite literally* the part of her that has kept her going-on-being through this horrific ordeal. This non-recognition, this disavowal by her father rendering Joy and Jack invisible, is enraging—and even beyond that, *shattering* to Joy.

Then, to Jack's horror, Joy makes a serious suicide attempt, slitting her wrists, draining the lifeblood from her body. It's Jack who finds her, saves her. Yet again. He is beside himself, terrified of losing her, and furious with her for abandoning him when she is hospitalized for several days, their first separation. When Joy comes home, Jack's terror and rage finally break through her dissociation, wake her up! to the catastrophe that losing her—his lifeline—would cause him, wake her up! to the singular importance of her existence for his. She tearfully apologizes to Jack in her old bedroom, a room which has not changed in the seven years Joy was missing. Her parents have kept her room frozen in time. Joy is devastated by all she has lost. Jack reaches out to touch her breast, asking, "Can I?," referring to breastfeeding. Joy replies tonelessly, in a semi-dissociated state, "There's no more left. Sorry." Then she starts to cry. She says, "I'm not a good enough mom." Without missing a beat, Jack responds, "But you're Ma!" And Joy laughs through her tears. "I am. I am."

But how do we understand Joy's attempted suicide given her fierce, all-consuming love and protectiveness of Jack? She could not hold Jack in mind, and the impact her suicide would have on him, in her dissociated, suicidal state, as the loving, responsible part of her was so split-off from the despairing, self-destructive self-state, similarly to Jack in chapter 2. For seven long years, she desperately dreamed of being rescued from imprisonment, of being back home with her family. But, in her father's disavowal of her existence, and of her present maternal self, which includes years of sexual violation and the creation of her son, Joy feels discarded, erased. Gerson's notion of a "dead third" comes to mind.

Who is Joy punishing in her suicide attempt? Her father, Jack? Is there also an internalization of Old Nick, who has become a dissociated part of Joy, that she is trying to kill off, Ferenczi's identification of the aggressor as a means of surviving massive trauma? Her suicide attempt is also an internalization of her father in his refusal to recognize Jack's existence, which then becomes an intergenerational repetition of her own traumatic experience of feeling erased, first by Old Nick, then by her father. And although Joy tried her best to protect Jack from her gruesome nightmare, we can wonder, if we view Jack as the patient, what seeped through, what did he witness, absorb, and carry with him of Joy's hopelessness, anguish, rage, and internalized violence? He is frequently put in the role of her protector, her rescuer. We, the audience, become Jack's witness.

Salberg and Grand (2017) speak to the complexity of role reversal in certain traumatic situations, where for various reasons, children end up caring for their parents, which both puts them at risk and potentially engenders resilience:

> The matching and tuning "dance" done by the child is often what attachment researchers like Lyons-Ruth (2002, 2003) consider a form of role reversal—that is, the child is attempting to affectively regulate the parent in lieu of the parent regulating the child ... This will become the *texture of traumatic attachment*—how it feels to this child to feel connected to the parent ... This may also be the place in which the child grows a kind of resilience, since in role reversal, the child is called upon to grow up sooner and to be, in a precocious manner, the more affectively regulated one.

In *The Body Keeps the Score,* Bessel Van der Kolk's (2014) classic text on the impact and healing of trauma, he describes a five-year-old's response to September 11, a little boy who witnessed the first plane slam into the World Trade Center from his classroom window. He witnessed people jumping from the towers, and then ran with his father and brother through the burning, smoking streets of lower Manhattan. The next day, the boy drew a picture of what he had witnessed the day before, but there was a little black circle at the foot of the buildings. When Van der Kolk asked him what that was, the little boy responded, "A trampoline, so that the next time when people have to jump, they will be safe." As Van der Kolk suggests, "This five-year old boy, a witness to unspeakable mayhem and disaster just twenty-four hours before he made that drawing, had used his imagination to process what he had seen and begin to go on with his life" (p. 52). Van der Kolk notes that his experience illustrates

> two crucial aspects of the adaptive response to threat that is basic to human survival ... He was able to take an active role by

running away, thus becoming an agent in his own rescue, and once he reached the safety of home, the alarm bells in his brain and body quieted. This freed his mind to make sense of what had happened and even to imagine a creative alternative to what he had seen—a life-saving trampoline (p. 53).

Jack too was an agent in his own rescue, but what a terrifying experience it was for him. Jack also had an expansive imagination and inner life that allowed him to manage Joy's periods of deadness and collapse. But what about the impact on Jack of being Joy's sole witness of her ongoing trauma, the burden imposed on Jack from birth. He seems so resilient but what about the burden on him as witness for his mom, as all she had that was good and real? How does Jack adapt to Joy's presences and absences, and especially to her "deadness?" Where does all that live in Jack? He was also the product of rape. How does Joy come to terms with that reality; or simply dissociate it (Solomon, 2012)? In Joy's serious suicide attempt, is there too an erasure, an attempt to erase all of the trauma: the kidnapping, the nightly rapes, the pregnancy, and even motherhood? The burden was just too great.

When I presented this paper at Division 39 in New York City in April 2018, the day before I presented it, it suddenly hit me that I was being too harsh with Joy's parents, that I was not empathizing enough with them. I had not been able to imagine my way into their inner worlds, into their overwhelming trauma. It suddenly hit me that, as a parent, it was *just too much*, too overwhelming to identify with Joy's parents, to imagine this traumatic story from *their* perspective. The enormous pain and shame of a father who did not—could not – protect his daughter from being abducted and raped, or bear Joy's suffering, who literally could not face her and her son; and a mother who struggled to hold onto hope that her daughter was alive seven years later, and the guilt of their marriage falling apart as a result.

Particularly in this volatile political moment, in the context of the #MeToo and #Time'sUp movements, the film can also be read from a feminist, sociopolitical perspective, speaking to issues of gender, sexuality, power, and powerlessness. We can explore the film in terms of rape culture, a culture rife with sexual violence and objectification. And what happens AFTER rape and sexual violence? There is often a lack of family and community support, an assumption that the woman did something to deserve it, an examination of how she dressed or her sexual history. Stigmatization leading to guilt and shame, and an avoidance of facing the horror. Joy's parents have difficulty understanding the depths of her traumatic experience. But they have been deeply traumatized as well, by the kidnapping and rape of their child, missing all that time, not knowing if they should keep hoping, not knowing if she was alive or dead.

So, reconsidering Viktor Frankl's central idea about the crucial importance of searching for meaning, even under the harshest conditions, what happens after the crisis is over, when Joy and Jack are freed from Room, when survivors are freed from torture, concentration camps, solitary confinement or death row? Sometimes, the extreme effort of surviving the trauma is, in a sense, containing, when one's only concern is how to make it *through*, to find creative means of staying enlivened when locked in an endless present. But, the aftermath can feel like an abyss. As psychoanalysts, how do we reckon with *all this trauma*? How do we provide a new "room" that contains the trauma, and allows the reliving of it, this time with us, as analysts and witnesses? Robert Jay Lifton (2017) suggests that healing from atrocity, from extreme trauma "seems to require a combination of confrontation and meaning-making in the death encounter, and at the same time moving beyond the death encounter into some dimension of renewal (p. 174)."

Dori Laub (2017a) writes about the crucial role of witnessing in trauma. He writes:

> Trauma, when re-lived and re-experienced in the context of a dialogue with an empathic listener, may restore to a degree, the victim's sense of being at home in the world. There's no longer the utter aloneness and incommunicability that's part of the extreme traumatic experience.

And sometimes a community can serve as a witness to mitigate the aloneness and incommunicability of a family's traumatic grief. When I presented an earlier version of this paper to the Tampa Bay Psychoanalytic Society in November 2018, something extraordinary occurred in the discussion afterward. Several people in the audience shared personal and professional stories of reckoning with and surviving severe trauma. Toward the end of the discussion, a woman stood up and shared a devastating story, truly every parent's worst nightmare. I wrote earlier that I realized belatedly that I had not been able to imagine my way into Joy's parents' worlds, because for me it was just too overwhelming to imagine the story from Joy's parents' perspective. And yet. This woman stood up and told us that 40 years ago, the unimaginable happened to her family. Her 11-year-old son was riding his bike to the candy store, and he was abducted, mutilated, and murdered. There was a collective gasp, and she went on to describe aspects of the still unfolding intergenerational transmission of this trauma to her children and grandchildren. Some of her colleagues knew, most didn't—she had never shared her story publicly before. I thanked her for her courage, and expressed my deep sorrow, and she left soon after the presentation.

I wrote to her the next day to thank her for sharing her heartbreaking story with us, and to let her know that she was heard and appreciated by all present, and that it touched me deeply. She sent me a beautiful note along with a copy of a memoir written by her youngest son, now a journalist, called *Alligator Candy*. Alligator Candy was the candy that this son, the author, had asked his older brother to buy for him at the candy store the last time he saw him, riding away on his red bike.

This story adds yet another layer of transformative resonance across multiple relational realms, and the power of witnessing to this story, themes I have been exploring in my writing for the past ten years. It also speaks to the ongoing challenges of a family struggling to find creative means of staying enlivened in the face of unspeakable trauma. Writing can be a vital part of that process. And witnessing can make the unbearable, vitally symbolizable, and communicable.

As analysts and witnesses, we must imagine our way into each other's worlds, allow ourselves to absorb the impact without flinching. Finding a way of witnessing without co-opting the other's subjectivity, knowing without colonizing (Levinas, 1969), can be both essential and daunting. These are the challenges of working with massive trauma, the crucial importance, and the challenges of allowing oneself to be deeply affected, risking vicarious traumatization. The inevitable wounding—and the transformative potential—of mutual vulnerability (Levine, 2016). But in this mutual survival of destructiveness and shame, there's also potentially a reaching toward reparation and mutual recognition.

In one of the most powerful passages of *Just Mercy*, Bryan Stevenson writes about brokenness and healing. He writes: "Being close to suffering, death, executions, and cruel punishments didn't just illuminate the brokenness of others; it also exposed my own brokenness." He says,

> We are all broken by something. We all share the condition of brokenness even if our brokenness is not equivalent. However, our brokenness is also the source of our common humanity, the basis for our shared search for comfort, meaning, and healing. Our shared vulnerability and our imperfection nurtures and sustains our capacity for compassion (p. 289).

Stevenson speaks to brokenness as both a wounding and, in essence, a state of grace (Dowd, 2016), holding the possibility, the hope, of renewal. A way of *listening and witnessing*, echoing Harris' notion that, as analysts, our *wounds must serve as tools*. I believe it's the essence of what makes change and transformation possible.

References

Bakewell, S. (2016). *At the existential café: Freedom, being, and apricot cocktails*. New York: Other Press.

Dowd, D. (2016). States of grace: A relational context for a patient's coming into being. *Psychoanalytic Dialogues*, 26: 564–570.

Frankl, V. (1959). *Man's search for meaning*. Boston: Beacon Press.

Gerson, S. (2009). When the third is dead: Memory, mourning and witnessing in the aftermath of the Holocaust. *International Journal of Psychoanalysis*, 90: 1341–1357.

Harris, A., & Bartlett, R. (2016). A window in time. *Psychoanalytic Dialogues*, 26, 129–135.

Laplanche, J. (1990). Implantation, intromission. In J. Fletcher (Ed.) *Essays on Otherness*, London: Routledge, 1999, 133–137.

Laub, D. (2017a). Reestablishing the internal "Thou" in testimony of trauma. In J. Alpert and E. Goren (Eds.) *Psychoanalysis, trauma and community: History and contemporary reappraisals*. London: Routledge.

Laub, D. (2017b). Listening to my mother's testimony. In J. Salberg and S. Grand (Eds.) *Wounds of history: Repair and resilience in the trans-generational transmission of trauma*. New York: Routledge.

Levinas, E. (1969). *Totality and infinity*. Pittsburgh: Duquesne University Press.

Levine, L. (2016). Mutual vulnerability: Intimacy, violation, and the shards of trauma. *Psychoanalytic Dialogues*, 26: 571–579.

Levine, L. (2018). Pina Bausch and the interweaving of trauma, memory and creative transformation: Discussion of Sarah Mendelsohn and Deborah Dowd's papers. *Psychoanalytic Dialogues*, 28: 94–101.

Lifton, R.J. (2017). The analyst as witness, historian, and activist: A conversation with E. Goren and J. Alpert (Eds) *Psychoanalysis, Trauma, and Community: History and contemporary reappraisals*. New York: Routledge.

Salberg, J. (2015). The texture of traumatic attachment: Presence and ghostly absence in transgenerational transmission. *Psychoanalytic Quarterly*, Vol. LXXXIV, 1: 21–46.

Salberg, J. and Grand, S. (2017). *Wounds of history: Repair and resilience in the trans-generational transmission of trauma*. New York: Routledge.

Scarfone, D. (2017). Ten short essays on how trauma is inextricably woven into psychic life. *Psychoanalytic Quarterly*, LXXXVI: 21–43.

Solomon, A. (2012). *Far from the tree: Parent, children and the search for identity*. New York: Scribner.

Stevenson, B. (2014). *Just mercy: A story of justice and redemption*. New York: Random House.

van der Kolk, B. (2014). *The body keeps the score: Brain, mind and body in the healing of trauma*. New York: Penguin.

Chapter 7

Becoming the Storyteller of One's Own Life

In her book, *The Faraway Nearby*, Rebecca Solnit (2013) writes about the vital importance and transformative potential of stories and storytelling, the ways in which stories can ground us, locate us, connect us, and imprison us. She writes:

> What's your story? Stories are compasses and architecture; we navigate by them, build our sanctuaries and our prisons out of them; and to be without a story is to be lost in the vastness of a world that spreads in all directions like arctic tundra or sea ice. To love someone is to put yourself in their place, which is to put yourself in their story ... Which means that a place is a story, and stories are geography; and empathy is first of all, an act of imagination, a storyteller's art ... A way of traveling from here to there (p. 1).

My patient, Darya, had lost the thread of her own story. She was once a dreamy little girl, a storyteller with a wondrous imagination. An only child who played alone in her room for hours, writing stories and creating imaginary worlds, Darya had big dreams. She dreamed of becoming a writer, an artist of one sort or another. Play and creativity served a crucial function for her, her imagination keeping her company, serving as a witness. But somewhere along the line, Darya got lost in the labyrinth of her immigrant parents' journey, imprisoned by their relational and intergenerational trauma, immobilized by their pressures, expectations, and sacrifices. She spoke tearfully of her fear of betraying Little Darya, of letting her down by not being true to her creative vision.

DOI: 10.4324/9781003367475-8

By the time she walked into my office, Darya was in her mid-twenties, depressed and panicked, suffering from an underlying existential dread. She was emotionally dysregulated, terrified of dying, anxious about multiple somatic complaints. I was struck by her intensity, her brilliance, creativity, and sense of humor—her abundant potential. And yet. Paralyzed by her parents' enigmatic messages (Laplanche and Pontalis, 1974), Darya felt profoundly stuck; she could not envision a psychic future (Cooper, 1997, 2016), and a sense of her own continuity, "a way of traveling from here to there." She could not sustain a sense of personal agency, as her life seemed characterized by doing and undoing, forward movement and backward undertow. Caught between divorced parents, a mother who fiercely assimilated and a father who refused to, and two worlds, her rich Lebanese heritage and her American identity, Darya could not live life in the present.

Darya seemed old before her time, anguished by the conundrum of having only one life to live. The poetry of Milan Kundera's, *The Unbearable Lightness of Being* came drifting back to me: "We can never know what to want, because living only one life, we can neither compare it with our previous lives, nor perfect it in our lives to come." Preoccupied by her favorite book, Ernest Becker's, *Denial of Death*, by mortality and the inherent meaninglessness of life, it was as if Darya were without a coherent narrative, without a compass, "lost in the vastness of a world that spreads in all directions like arctic tundra or sea ice."

In this chapter, I am going to explore the impact of intergenerational and migration trauma on the challenge of creating one's own coherent story—resonant with both personal authenticity and a shared sense of culture and history. In analysis, this entails engaging and bearing what Rozmarin (2018) calls, "the frontier between the subjective and the collective," engaging and bearing intrapsychic and intergenerational experiences of shame and illegitimacy and disrupting traumatic cycles. The backdrop of racial melancholia (Eng and Han, 2019) further complicates this process, interfering with what Seligman (2016) calls, becoming "a self in time," "a sense of personal security, vital intersubjectivity and temporality … a sense of moving forward into a lively future" (pp. 110–111).

As I wrote in Chapter Two, Seligman notes that a mother's attuned response to her infant's spontaneous gesture creates intersubjective communication and meaning, giving the baby "compelling evidence of her effect on the world." When a mother is not responsive to an infant's gestures, "there is no sense of time moving forward," only "the stasis of a present which never gives way to an emergent future." Far from being responsive to Darya's spontaneous gestures, Darya experienced her mother as controlling, depriving Darya of a sustained sense of her own agency and effectance. However, in Darya's mind, this was her immigrant mother's way of expressing love and concern, an effort to protect Darya from the trauma and anguish she went through in her own life, wanting a better life for Darya. I am going to expand on Seligman's seminal ideas, adding a transgenerational and sociocultural dimension (see Harris and Bartlett, 2015). I will interweave these cultural layers into my story with Darya, who was held captive by ghosts of relational trauma and melancholia (Eng and Han, 2000; Harris et al. 2016).

Gonzalez (2016) writes, "The displacement occasioned by immigration—especially when forced by political oppression or economic deprivation—is a tremendous challenge to subjectivity" (p. 15). But, "these migratory displacements are also the fertile ground of creativity, the strange place where something new can come into being." They are not only "the *wellsprings of grief*, they're also *the engines of poetry*" (p. 17). I want you to imagine yourself into Darya's existential ennui, her sense of being stuck in time, caught in the web of her immigrant parents' intergenerational trauma. But imagine too, her desperate longing to forge an identity of her own based on her own fantasies and desires, a deep need to find her voice, and create her own poetry. This is a story of Darya's struggle to become a self in time, to reclaim her creative agency, and become the storyteller of her own life.

In my work with Darya, I had the sense that she was carrying the weight of history, the anguish of past generations. While I described her initially as a dreamy little girl, a storyteller with a wondrous imagination, I came to understand that this was not the whole story. This idealized origin story was in part, Darya's fantasy of wholeness, a romanticized version of herself and her world before her parents' separation and divorce, dissociating the impact of her mother's narcissistic investment and control, and devoid of intergenerational trauma. This story has gaps and holes, "gaps left within her by the secrets of others" (Abraham, 1988). Harris (2016) asks, "What makes time stop, or rather, what allows *or requires* a person to step outside the flow of time and history, transmitting the past into the present? How is the experience of haunting so inexorably passed on from parent to child?" (p. 182). In his writing on transgenerational haunting, Abraham (1988) suggests that what haunts us are not *the dead*, but the gaps left within us by the secrets of others.

Though Darya was brilliant, creative, and full of potential, though she had powerful hopes and dreams, there was paradoxically also a palpable brokenness, a loneliness and fragmentation that she could not articulate and did not understand. She had frequent somatic ailments and a terror that something was very wrong in her body. I had the sense that there were ghosts hovering, haunting, holding her body and mind captive (Harris et al., 2016; Dowd, 2018), and that I would need to get to know those ghosts intimately, over time.

But what does it mean to "get to know a patient's ghosts in-timately?" I believe it entails being open to being haunted oneself, allowing in, and engaging with the ghosts of one's own past (Dowd, 2018; Harris, et al., 2016). There were times when Darya's embodied trauma, especially as expressed in her intense anxiety about multiple somatic complaints, and a terror that she was dying, felt so hard to sit with. In my efforts to immerse myself in her existential dread, I found myself caught up in her myriad somatic anxieties, which stirred intense anxieties in me. Several years before I began seeing Darya, my two younger sisters were diagnosed with breast cancer within two years of each other, during which time my mother died unexpectedly after an infection from an aortic valve replacement. Although both of my sisters are thankfully healthy, this collision of life-threatening family events left me feeling deeply vulnerable in terms of my own health, and destabilizingly face to face with my own mortality. I was aware of dreading/fighting/pro-testing facing my own mortality with open eyes. In Chapter Four, I wrote that mutual vulnerability "entails a willingness to be deeply unsettled and dysregulated by our most wounded patients." But I wonder how areas of deep vulnerability can also lead to dissociation in the analyst, and potentially, at least temporarily, get in the way of going deeper into the patient's wounds and unresolved traumas.

In retrospect, I think this dissociative dynamic played out in the writing of this chapter, although I did not become aware of it until I presented an earlier version of this paper. My sessions with Darya had almost always felt compelling and alive, even when she was plagued by existential weariness and a terror of dying and deadness. But I grappled in an ongoing way to capture this clinical aliveness in my writing. I struggled to write about my work with Darya in an experience-near way, and I kept feeling a sense of deadness in my writing. It was only after a presentation of this paper that I gave at the International Association of Relational Psychotherapy and Psychoanalysis (IARPP) in Los Angeles in 2022, our first conference after two years of death and dying and pandemic delays, that a colleague (Sandy Silverman, personal communication, June 2022) shared her insight that my struggle mirrored and enacted Darya's battle with aliveness and deadness, inspiration and creative blocks. This immediately resonated for me. Once I recognized this as a potential projective identification, a communication of Darya's struggle with aliveness and deadness, her fervent efforts to center creativity in her life, my writing started to flow. Once I was able to reflect on the "ghosts hovering, haunting, holding Darya's body and mind captive, and that I would need to get to know those ghosts intimately over time," I was able to open a door to my own affective experience, countertransference and creativity.

Building on Faimberg's notion of a telescoping of generations, Salberg (2015) suggests that it may take three generations to contain disturbing feelings and events. Unspoken traumatic stories and dissociated affect get passed from one generation to the next, as "parents extrude the traumatic contents of their minds into their children" (p. 78). This has echoes of Laplanchian enigmatic messages, a too-muchness that parents pass on unconsciously to their children. Darya was paralyzed by ungrieved loss and trauma from her intergenerational past. She had absorbed enigmatic and conflicting messages from her parents: the *burden of trauma* and the *burden of hope* from her immigrant parents. They had both experienced terror and violence in their early lives, the specifics of which were hazy to Darya. There was so much I did not know about Darya's parents and grandparents.

What I did know was this. Her parents, both immigrants from middle-class families in Lebanon, went in opposite directions settling here in the United States Her father, a laid back, creative designer, never assimilated in his 35 years in the U.S., and barely speaks English, though he is successful within his small Lebanese community. Darya speaks only Arabic with him. Darya loves and identifies with her father's creativity ("the sweetest, most creative person in the world"), but is also embarrassed and ashamed by his foreignness. Her mother, a successful businesswoman, who had had an emotionally and physically abusive father, threw herself into American culture, and had big dreams for Darya, her only daughter. But they were *her* dreams, infused by the losses *she* had suffered, by the opportunities *she* had not had.

Darya's parents, who had had an arranged marriage, separated when Darya was quite young. Darya continued living with her mother, but remembers her father visiting often, playing pretend play with her dolls, teaching her to ride a bike, and watching movies together at his apartment. She spent much time with her father's family, and remembers feeling uncomfortable, like she did not fit in with her cousins, who were less Americanized. She felt close to her mother, although their relationships was fraught, and Darya experienced her as domineering and critical, and in many ways, felt held hostage by her. Her father was more relaxed, but felt "more foreign," and less available, less known to her. She longed for more of him, more involvement and interest *from* him, and more of his laid-backness *in* her. Early on, I understood that Darya never felt truly seen or recognized by either parent for very different reasons, though she loved them both deeply.

Rachel Kabasakalian-McKay, in a discussion of my paper at the 2019 Stephen Mitchell Relational Center Conference, on Surviving Destruction, wrote that I begin my paper by citing Rebecca Solnit, who describes poetically how "stories locate us." Kabasakalian-McKay wonders about the ways in which my choice of an epigraph "reflects not only (Darya's) difficulty weaving a narrative for her own life, *but (my) longing to find aspects of Darya's experience that remain somehow out of reach as well as unformulated.*" This resonated powerfully for me in the gaps in my understanding of Darya and the impact of her parents' unprocessed, unformulated trauma.

In her discussion, Kabasakalian-McKay suggested that both Darya and I were "longing to repair a wound in an other whose dimensions she can't quite see." She suggested that I am trying to imagine and repair a wound in Darya, while Darya desperately seeks to imagine and heal unmourned, and not fully known trauma in her mother. This has echoes of Henri Rey (1988), building on Klein, who posits that patients come into treatment to repair their damaged inner objects, the wounds from prior generations.

Curiously, yet perhaps connected to these insights by Kabasakalian-McKay, Darya had always felt an intense, yet impossible pressure to answer life's existential questions *before living* her life. She was desperate to find a creative means of becoming enlivened, but each time she had a creative aspiration, her mother would criticize and undermine her, causing her to doubt herself and her choices. Pulled continually into a Winnicottian false-self position of compliance, she longed for authentic self-expression, but immediately doubted and denigrated her choices, instead of pursuing them more deeply, and seeing them through. She would get inspired, alight on an idea, but her choices never felt true or right. Unable to settle on a career or even a direction in life, Darya felt haunted by the ghost of "Childhood Darya," who called to her to be an artist, to live a creative life, a life of her choosing.

When we first met, Darya was halfway through graduate school at a prestigious university, a choice she had felt pressured into by her mother, who wanted her only child to have a stable, successful profession. She was an outstanding student, at the top of her class, yet strung out and miserable. Harshly self-critical and critical of others, she was ferociously competitive and driven, with herself and her classmates. She was determined to stand out, be the best, even as she was preoccupied by the idea of *dropping out.* Her mother was adamant that she finish graduate school and become a successful professional who could support herself, not be dependent on anyone to take care of her. Darya was torn. She longed to be in a creative field, wistful for her childhood state of wonder and awe, but felt guilty about how much her parents had sacrificed. And especially as an only child of immigrants, there was much unconscious pressure to contain the dislocation and trauma in both her parents' families, to fulfill her parents' dreams and expectations.

From the beginning, I was struck by the many splits and binaries in Darya's thinking, sense of self, and ways of being. She could be both grandiose, and ruthlessly self-critical. She felt so much pressure; a sense that she was destined to do great things, but felt she could not possibly live up to those perfectionistic ideals. Moderation, compromise, "good enough" were not an option. She either had to be the best, be first in her class, in every class, or opt out, drop out, move far away from the demands of big city East coast life, where she fantasized she could just live in the moment. Ambitious and aggressive like her mother, creative like her father. This split, the hard driving, critical, perfectionist mom and the laid-back, creative dad were at war in Darya's mind when she arrived in my office at 25, depressed, anxious, somatic, and unable to settle on any decision about what direction to go in her life. Without a compass. Decisions, coherence, any movement felt illusive.

Stephen Mitchell's notions of psychopathology as stasis feel relevant here. In one of his classic papers, Penelope's Loom, Mitchell wrote: "Psychopathology reflects our unconscious commitment to stasis, to stuckness, embeddedness in and loyalty to the familiar." You can hear the influence of Loewald and Fairbairn in the repetition of old patterns and dynamics, fidelity to old objects, to the past, to the familiar. Harris (2009, 2010) writes about mourning as a prerequisite to growth and change and omnipotence as a defense against mourning. Splitting disrupts mourning; it prolongs melancholia. Darya was trapped in impossible splits in the service of melancholia, by wanting everything, unable to make a decision or accept any limitations. She was unable to integrate multiple identifications and cultural identities. If she chose to identify with one parent, if she moved toward one identification, then she felt she was betraying the other, and there was irreparable loss. The developmental work of mourning and integration felt daunting. Why was mourning so unbearable?

Darya's mother was the first woman in her family to get a college and then graduate school education. She was fiercely determined to be successful, and resolute that her only daughter should follow in her footsteps. For Darya, along with the intergenerational trauma haunting her family, there was also a pull for intergenerational continuity, a feminist pride in her mother's struggles and accomplishments. A drive for success, and enormous respect for how hard her mother fought to free herself from her traumatic past to establish herself as an independent woman in the U.S. Darya was conscious of the freedom and opportunities she had had as a woman growing up in the U.S. that her mother and grandmothers had not had in

Lebanon. She felt guilty about her difficulty launching herself into adulthood, given the privileges she had been afforded, but this guilt was stultifying rather than mobilizing.

Her mother's fraught warning hung over her: This is what you could/ could not have been as a woman growing up in Lebanon when I was growing up. America offered the promise of opportunity, new and better economic choices, which Darya recognized and consciously appreciated. She identified as American, as a New Yorker, but in some unconscious realm, was she operating as if she were stuck in time, back in Lebanon in a past generation? Darya was painfully aware of her mother's desperate desire to protect her from the myriad traumas and struggles she herself had suffered. But there was a too-muchness in her relationship with her mother, and the line between protection and colonization felt precarious, porous, easily breached. Her mother was so critical of her only child, now a young adult struggling to free herself from her mother's projections, and from the critical internal objects in her head. Though she had always considered her relationship with her mother to be "close," though conflictual, Darya and I came to understand the ways in which her mother's narcissistic investment and appropriation served as a barrier to following her heart, trusting her own voice, and her own desires, leaving her feeling empty and overwhelmed.

I was attentive, in my work with Darya, to our cultural differences. I tried to be aware of my own biases, as a White, Jewish American professional woman having grown up in the U.S., where values of separation/ individuation are woven into the American ethos, and into our psychoanalytic and developmental theories. I am the granddaughter, not the daughter of Eastern European immigrants. My upper middle class parents encouraged me to follow my dreams. Was Darya ever told to follow her dreams? I was mindful of the importance for Darya of gratitude, loyalty, and a deep connection to her parents; a powerful, emotional awareness of their struggles, and the value of family loyalty in Lebanese culture.

But Darya was conflicted about her cultural identity. In some ways, she disowned her Lebanese background. She saw herself as White, which she says is how her mom raised her. She valued her American culture, or more precisely, her New York culture, her chosen home, the life she *chose*, as opposed to the life of her ancestors. Darya didn't want to see herself or be seen as Other, to be coded as Other, and she enjoyed the privileges of passing as White. She told me she was "not interested" in what happened generations before her, that it wasn't "interesting" to her. Many of the details of her parents' traumatic migration histories were fuzzy to her. But there were cracks in this narrative. Darya became tearful *whenever* she talked about her parents' anguish leaving their homeland, the trauma they experienced in the violent civil war, and their grief and wistfulness about the life and culture they left behind. Whose tears was she shedding? Although she identified as a New Yorker and denied being "interested" in her culture of origin, the intergenerational trauma leaked through. Her tears betrayed her.

This disconnection from history, this severing of her family's migration story, the fantasy that one can be whole outside history, makes the developmental work of mourning and integration enormously challenging. I wondered, could this splitting off of her Lebanese identity, racial melancholia, be an aspect of Darya's depression and somatization, which Eng and Han (2000) allude to as intergenerational and cultural "dis-ease"? (p. 684). Was Darya's paralysis and somatization a form of melancholic sacrifice and racial dissociation? (Eng and Han, 2000). Eng and Han write about the erasure of cultural trauma, registering transgenerational cultural trauma in the body. They write:

> In melancholia, the subject's turning from outside (intersubjective) to inside (intrapsychic) threatens to render the social invisible … The daughters' bodies and voices become substitutes for those of the mothers—not just the mothers' bodies and voices, but also something that is unconsciously lost in them (p. 683).

Eng and Han suggest that "sacrifice is built on the melancholic notion that what is forfeited and lost can never be recuperated." They ask, "Do children of immigrants "repay" this sacrifice only by repeating and perpetuating its melancholic logic—by berating and sacrificing themselves?" (p. 681).

Maurice Apprey (2014) writes about the *pluperfect errand of the unconscious in transgenerational haunting.* It's an errand because it lies in reserve waiting to happen, and *a pluperfect errand because it's a parental project related to unresolved trauma and mourning that has already happened but was only lying in wait for its messenger(s).*

One generation sends an urgent message to the next, but it's an impossible mission that cannot be fulfilled because it's not of this time, this generation. Darya's desire to "pass" as White, as a White American is an aspect of Apprey's pluperfect errand. What was the melancholic price of passing White?

For a child of immigrants, creating one's own origin story, a differentiated narrative can feel like an abandonment—a betrayal of her parents' sacrifices, the tie to their cultural heritage. But a fear of abandoning her parents left Darya caught in a bind and a betrayal of her own lived experience. Darya had to locate, or actually construct her own narrative in the architecture of her lived experience, in order to find her place in her parents' ancestral story. How complicated to forge an identity that integrated her American and Lebanese cultures, especially with the split between her parents, one who longed for assimilation, and one who dreaded dislocation from his country and culture.

I wonder how Darya's family's traumatic migration story and her cultural identity struggles informed her complex, nonlinear journey to becoming an artist, or at least, living a creative life. Edwidge Danticat (2011) writes, in *Create Dangerously: The Immigrant Artist at Work,* writes:

> The immigrant artist must quantify the price of the American dream in flesh and bone. All this while living with the more *regular* fears of any other artist. Do I know enough about where I've come from? Will I ever know enough about where I am? Even if somebody has died for me to stay here, will I ever truly belong? (pp. 17–18)

Darya felt so indebted to her parents, so aware of how much they had sacrificed, but this indebtedness stifled her. Over time, she was able to get more in touch with her rage toward her mother for her control and criticism, and aware of the degree of their enmeshment and her compliance. It has been a challenge to separate her appreciation and gratitude for being part of a legacy of strong women from being entitled to have a life of her own choosing, a voice of her own. As she gradually began to separate from her mother, she began to stand up to her more, to speak her mind, assert her desire and opinions. This was a huge step, and Darya had much trepidation, confronting her mother, managing her mother's anger and disappointment. But her efforts to separate and individuate from her mother did not vanquish the ruthless, harshly self-critical internalized voices in her head, Fairbairn's internal saboteur.

While Darya had a more conflictual relationship with her mother, she longed to know and be known more by her father, whom she saw as the creative one, the one who put less pressure on her, who encouraged her to pursue her dreams. But he was harder for her to relate to, as she resented his refusal to assimilate, to learn English and more about American culture. Darya felt ashamed of his foreignness, even as she yearned to be seen and recognized by him. Several years into therapy, as she had spoken tearfully about her desire to be closer to him, she had an inspired idea: to design and build a cottage with him, a joint creative venture. The fantasy did not involve *living* in the cottage; the importance was in the *building*, the learning from her father and communicating with him in his own language, a joint language, the language of architecture and design. And the sharing of their creative aesthetics. Solnit again: "A place is a story, and stories are geography." We talked about this as an attempt to locate herself in the world, and in her father's mind and heart. And perhaps a fantasy of transference-countertransference with me in the cottage, in the consulting room, no longer alone in her childhood bedroom, a fantasy of building something together?

Weeks later, Darya told me that she had spent an hour with both parents. She became teary when she talked about how "cute" they were, how well they get along now, and how she imagined the life she could have had if they had stayed together. "Three is so much better than two," she said tearfully, sounding like the Little Darya I imagined in my mind. She told me they were meeting together because she was going ahead with the building of the cabin, which her dad had designed architecturally, and now her mom was going to be the project manager. We talked about how poignant this was, the three of them building a cottage, a home together–her idea, her conception, her fantasy that she was making come true. And yet, soon afterward, the idealized bubble popped. She told me: "I had my first fight with my dad in years last week. He said he wanted to arrange a marriage for me with a Lebanese guy, even though I'm engaged to Jason. He's so foreign. I can't believe that's my dad!!" While Darya can get caught up in her fantasies of family wholeness and integration, the splits and barriers to psychic integration still loom large.

Over the course of our work together, as Darya developed more of a sense of personal agency, and found her own voice, as she felt more grounded in herself, she also felt freer to appreciate her Lebanese culture, which she had often repudiated, and disowned. She planned a creative Lebanese dinner for friends that she prepared and cooked, with recipes from her mom, who learned them from her mom, who was, of course, delighted.

Darya gradually allowed me to enter the arctic tundra of her psychic landscape, to imagine my way into her melancholic world. Gerson suggests, "The mutual creation of coherence alters the private and dark unknown of the individual unconscious into a shared geography of meaning" (p. 93). Through our work together, we are developing a shared geography of meaning, as Darya is beginning to feel less alone, more embodied, less somatic, more connected to her intergenerational history, and more enlivened.

In the middle of her last year of grad school, having separated more from her mother, Darya made the radical decision not to pursue a career in that field, a courageous statement of her commitment to move into a creative field, and out of a compliant position with her mother, who was, not surprisingly, quite upset by this decision. More confident articulating and valuing her own creative voice, she found an internship in a film company, to the surprise of her friends, family, and professors. But when the internship ended, Darya spent several months feeling depressed, anxious and immobilized, wracked by doubts about whether she had made the wrong decision. Stuck once again.

During our work together, I was simultaneously working on the paper that became Chapter Six, about the film, *Room*. While Darya was not imprisoned in a room, nevertheless she felt imprisoned by her own mind, trapped and stuck in an endless present, unable to move forward in her life. I have written about reverberations across multiple relational realms, how reveries from other treatments, supervisions, and papers come unbidden into our writing and work with patients. Like my patient Julia, in Chapter Two, Darya had periods of creative expansiveness, but her attempts at creative means of staying enlivened kept coming to a screeching halt when she inevitably denigrated each initially inspiring creative foray. Every time she took a creative leap forward, the critical internalized maternal voices would come rushing in, leaving Darya feeling hopeless and despairing. Caught in her melancholy about Little Darya, a romantic nostalgia for an earlier time with the illusion of wholeness—of identity, family structure, cultural integration, a Laplanchian re-transcribing of traumatic experience, après coup.

Darya perpetually felt as if she were running out of time, which seeped into our work together. I wondered: Was this urgency, anxiety, fear of running out of time; this breathless, dissociated panic on some level echoing her parents' flight from Lebanon? She came to each session with a sense of urgency, and *anxiety*, sometimes with a list of things to talk about on her phone, as if there was not enough time to share *everything* on her mind with me. On one hand, this felt like a way of controlling the flow of sessions, not allowing herself to be fully immersed and present, but I also wondered whether this came from a fierce desire to make order and sense out of the compartmentalized and disjunctive stories in her mind. I also felt her sense of desperation to not forget anything, to tell me everything. I often slowed her down, encouraged her to breathe, asked her to pay attention to what she was feeling in her body. At times she felt frustrated by not getting through her list. But often she appreciated my helping her to feel less dysregulated, more embodied, and more present with me in the room. At times, this allowed for more connection and mutual recognition, creating a sense of creativity and flow in the analysis. Our work together in the Room, in the cottage, helped Darya begin to gain some traction, agency, and intentionality, a nascent sense of herself in time (Seligman, 2016).

A couple of years ago, Darya brought up termination, or at least "a break" from therapy for the first time. She said she felt like she had "met her goals," and marveled at how much had changed. And much had changed. Darya said,

I'm living my life, I'm IN my life. I feel more present, not constantly questioning, less perfectionistic. I've found a job I actually love. I'm much more separate from my mom, both in our relationship, and in my mind. I can roll my eyes when she makes a critical, undermining comment about my new career, rather than feeling devastated.

"But," then a sharp shift in self-states as she worriedly asked, "how do we do this, how do we take a break from therapy? Is it going to feel like ripping away my blanket?" I heard Little Darya asking me plaintively. Help me grow up, help me separate from you lovingly, in a way that doesn't hurt, in a way I wish my mother could do for me. I felt conflicted. Darya had grown significantly in many ways and was more in touch with her own desires and how to act on them. She no longer had significant somatic ailments or a foreboding, all-encompassing existential ennui. But she still struggled enormously to bring her desires into fruition, to feel content and satisfied with her choices, as the violent undertow of doubt tortured her, making forward momentum enormously challenging.

So, Darya and I talked about taking a break from therapy. Looking back on this, I wondered whether perhaps she needed to "kill me off" to go forward in her life, a Loewaldian parricide. I had just started working on writing this paper and had asked her permission to write about her. Where did that live in her decision to "take a break?" She seemed, in fact, delighted that I was that interested in her, invested in her, that I wanted to spend so much time reflecting on her and our work together. I read her the first few paragraphs, and tears ran down her face, just as they did when she talked about her parents' history and their angst leaving Lebanon. Leaving, escaping, becoming. Darya told me that what I had written resonated for her, and she was eager to read the paper when it was finished.

Six months later, Darya emailed me to come back to therapy. She told me about her new entrepreneurial idea, about which she had been thrilled and delighted, but how she always gets "bored," self-doubting and self-critical. Familiar territory.

Darya: "It gets to a point where I just want to "escape" from a project. I'm totally stressed out. I can't sleep or eat well or take care of myself. All I do is work. I feel so unfree. I keep building prisons."

I hear Solnit again, "Stories are compasses and architecture; we navigate by them, build our sanctuaries and our prisons out of them."

Me: "Building prisons?"

Darya described her pattern of getting inspired and excited, but then driving herself so intensely that she exhausts herself, feeling like the only way out is to quit. I asked about earlier memories of feeling unfree. She shared, for the first time: "My mom forced me to do all these things she thought an American girl should do, like go to overnight camp. I felt trapped, homesick. I cried so much till my mom let me leave. I had to get so despondent to get permission to leave."

Me:	"It still feels that way, that you need to get so despondent, so tortured and bottomed out to get permission, to give *yourself* permission to be released from prison."
Darya:	"Yes."

A few sessions later, Darya came in worried about telling her mom something that would upset her. I asked: "How do you feel about upsetting her, about her being sad or disappointed?"

Darya:	"Awful! It's the worst thing ever. I just want her to make her happy. The thought of upsetting her is so upsetting to me. Her influence on me is so, so much less than it was. But I still hate making her sad. It's still hurtful that she doesn't approve of anything I do." Then a dramatic shift in self-states. "She's so loving and nurturing." I must have looked surprised. "Well, she doesn't realize how hurtful her control and criticism are, and she doesn't do it on purpose. She did the best she could. She's a supermom in so many ways." Long pause. "But I'd trade that for a person I could call with a problem and have her talk me through it." Darya looked very sad. "She really doesn't know me at all."

Each time Darya took a step forward, embracing her desire and building on her dreams, she inevitably found herself struggling with a new conundrum that relied again on splitting. Shifting back into old dynamics with her mother, back into a paranoid/schizoid position, keeping her stuck in time, trapped in impossible splits in the service of melancholia, unable to make a decision or accept any limitations.

Because choosing—like growth and change, entails loss, and she still struggles to bear loss, to mourn. And the splits in her Lebanese/American identity still felt fractured, dissociated.

Danticat's words rang in my ears: The immigrant artist must quantify the price of the American dream in flesh and bone.

We worked together for another few months, but just when I sensed our work deepening, when Darya seemed more able to tolerate conflict and ambiguity, to begin to mourn the past and make decisions about the future, Darya announced that she was ready to take a break again. I challenged her, encouraged her to reflect on our starts and stops as a repetition, reflective of the central issue we have been working on throughout our time together. I wondered what she may be avoiding in terms of a deeper, more vulnerable relationship, concerns about dependency, or my colonization or control? I had the feeling that Darya humored me, but was determined to stick with her decision to leave.

I imagine that Darya will reappear, that she and I are still in transit, still struggling, and that we will continue to process the sociocultural trauma passed on to her, work on living in the in-between places, the liminal spaces. She is less plagued by existential dread and somatic ailments, and more able to reflect on her tendency to split, as well as the limitations of binary thinking. She is less dissociated and more present, in a happy, stable relationship with someone who understands and treasures her, and with whom she shares a creative mind.

Davies (1999) makes the point that we must be willing to risk getting lost with our patients, as otherwise, there is little depth, therapeutic action, or creativity in the treatment. She writes:

> The analyst must be prepared ... to feel lost and out of control, to sometimes 'wander' in an effort to find herself again. Indeed, if we do not lose ourselves along the way, we will conduct a trip in which we see only the known and familiar spots. We will never happen upon those special moments of unexpected delight hidden off the beaten track (pp. 205–206).

Traveling from here to there with our patients requires acts of courage and imagination, as well as a willingless to get lost, to live in the messy unknown, Navigating the stark landscape of arctic tundra and sea ice where growth is hard to come by in the frozen soil. This journey can be treacherous, far from linear. But add to this, the weight of history, the impact and complexity of intergenerational and cultural trauma, and these stories we tell ourselves become that much more challenging to rewrite, to create poetry out of the "gaps left within us by the secrets of others (Abraham, 1988)."

References

Abraham, N. (1988). Notes on the phantom. In F. Meltzer (Ed.) *The trials of psychoanalysis* (p. 75–80). Chicago, University of Chicago Press.

Apprey, M. (2014). A pluperfect errand: A turbulent return to beginnings in the transgenerational transmission of destructive aggression. *Free Associations*, 15:16–29.

Cooper, S. H. (2016). Mourning, regeneration, and the psychic future: A discussion of Levine's "A mutual survival of destructiveness and its creative potential for agency and desire". *Psychoanal. Dialogues*, 26:56–62. 10.1080/10481885.2016.1123517.

Danticat, E. (2011). *Create dangerously: The immigrant artist at work.* New York: Vintage Books.

Davies, J. (1999). Getting cold feet, defining "safe-enough" borders: dissociation, multiplicity, and integration in the analyst's experience. *Psychoanal. Q.*, 68:184–208.

Dowd, D. (2018). The unfreezing of time in the haunted hours. *Psychoanal. Dialogues*, 28:69–77.

Eng, D. and Han, S. (2000). A dialogue on racial melancholia. *Psychoanalytic Dialogues*, 10: 667–700.

Eng, D. and Han, S. (2019). *Racial melancholia, racial dissociation: On the social and psychic lives of Asian Americans.* Durham: Duke University Press.

Gonzalez, F. (2016). Only what is human can truly be foreign: The trope of immigration as a creative force in psychoanalysis. In J. Beltsiou (Ed.) *Immigration in psychoanalysis.* London: Routledge.

Harris, A. (2010). The analyst's omnipotence and the analyst's melancholy.

Harris, A., and Bartlett, R. (2015). A window in time: A response to "disorders of temporality and the subjective experience of time: Unresponsive objects and the vacuity of the future" by Stephen Seligman. *Psychoanal. Dialogues*, 26:129–135. 10.1080/10481885.2016.1144956.

Harris, A. Kalb, M , and Klebanoff, S. (Eds.) (2016). First kiss, last word: Stairway to heaven. In *Ghosts in the consulting room: Echoes of trauma in psychoanalysis.* London: Routledge.

Laplanche, J. & Pontalis, J. (1974). *The language of psychoanalysis*. London: The Hogarth Press.

Rey, J.H. (1988). That which patients bring to analysis. *Int J Psychoanal.* 69: 457–470.

Rozmarin, E. (2018). Silence=Death, Co-Constructing Silence/Co-Constructing Voice. Institute for Contemporary Psychotherapy Conference, October 2018.

Salberg, J. (2015). The texture of traumatic attachment: Presence and ghostly absence in transgenerational transmission. *Psychoanal. Q.*, 84, 21–46. 10.1002/j.2167-4086.2015.00002.x.

Seligman, S. (2016). Disorders of temporality and the subjective experience of time: Unresponsive objects and the vacuity of the future. *Psychoanalytic Dialogues*, 26: 110–128.

Solnit, R. (2013). *The faraway nearby*. New York: Penguin Books.

Chapter 8

Interrogating Race, Shame, and Mutual Vulnerability in Psychoanalysis

I began writing this chapter in the spring of 2020, during a cataclysmic collision of the COVID-19 pandemic and a long overdue White awakening to the pandemic of anti-Black racism, police violence, and racial trauma in the U.S. The pandemic disproportionately afflicted Black, Indigenous, Asian Americans, and other people of color, laying bare long-standing socioeconomic and racial inequities at the heart of American life. This White reckoning with the structural and institutional racism embedded in American history, culture, and politics was triggered by the murder of George Floyd, a Black man, by Derek Chauvin, a White Minneapolis cop. One of innumerable acts of anti-Black police violence, the cellphone video of George Floyd's brutal murder and his desperate cries of *I can't breathe* echoed around the world, breaking through the dissociation and opening the eyes of some White Americans.

I start from the premise that America is haunted by our shameful history of chattel slavery and the slaughter and displacement of Indigenous people, and that we must find a way to acknowledge and grapple with what Nichols and Connolly (2020) call, the *moral injury,* at the heart of our nation's history. Whether we acknowledge it or not, we are all "implicated" in the iniquitous history of our nation (Rothberg, 2019; Kabasakalian-McKay and Mark, 2022; Gay, 2016), as *beneficiaries or descendants.* Nichols and Connolly (2020) assert, "No one escapes the taint of a crime against humanity" (p. 17). Do we, as psychoanalysts, teachers, supervisors, writers, and editors, have the moral stamina for an honest confrontation with the racist violence of our country's past and ongoing present, and the

DOI: 10.4324/9781003367475-9

internalized racism we carry within us? As James Baldwin reminds us: "The trouble is deeper than we realized because the trouble is in us."

My aim is to prompt reflection on what Harris (2019) calls *the perverse pact*; White America's dissociation of the narcissistic wound and collective trauma caused by the long arc of slavery, White supremacy and systemic racism, in our country and within psychoanalysis, and its scarring impact on Black, Brown, and White bodies and minds, *not equally, but nonetheless corrosively*. This entails facing ways in which White Americans have benefited from the institutionalization of White privilege and control. It demands of all of us a sense of responsibility, and an obligation to participate in the dismantling of racism, in the deconstructing and reconstruction of more equitable, anti-racist analytic spaces (Sadek, in press). I welcome Stephens' (2022) nuanced query in her discussion of this paper in *Psychoanalytic Dialogues*, related to issues of race, power, and caste (Wilkerson, 2020):

> The deeper implication Lauren Levine finds herself wrestling with in her consulting room, especially with her patients of color, is, what does it mean to think about relational racialization as a process that we are all subject to and subjected by, even if with more or less detrimental, corrosive effects on our senses of self?

I believe this requires a radical shift in our conception of the analytic frame, necessitating stepping outside of a familiar, comfortable role in which we have been taught to follow what patients bring to analysis; the analyst as the one who listens, makes space for the patient to speak. Rather than waiting for our patients to bring up issues of race, I believe it behooves White analysts to take the lead in listening for and speaking directly about race, racism and racial identity especially if they do not do so spontaneously, to make it clear that we are invested in, and up for these challenging discussions. Numerous analysts of color have described years of therapy with a White analyst, where race was never even mentioned. I believe this requires us to be open and curious, to interrogate our own and our patients' intersectional and intergenerational histories and identities, to ask about the wounds of racial, class, gender, and sexual trauma, experiences of otherness and being othered. Clearly this requires sensitivity, care, deep listening, and a willingness to take risks, get messy, make mistakes, try to repair racialized enactments when they inevitably occur, and, as Vaughans (2022) suggests in his discussion of this paper in *Psychoanalytic Dialogues*, to reach *out* rather than *down*, to "construct necessary scaffolding to bridge the divide" in cross-racial dyads. The question of, "What's it like for you to work with a White analyst?" is far from enough and will not serve to deepen the analysis without ongoing attention to and inquiry about race.

In her book, *Out of the Sun: On Race and Storytelling*, Esi Edugyan (2021) explores what it means to be seen, and who remains unseen. She asks: "What happens when we begin to consider stories at the margins, when we grant them centrality? How does that complicate our certainties about who we are, as individuals, as nations, as human beings?" She writes, "We must first acknowledge the vastly unequal places from which we each speak, the ways some have been denied voices when others are so easily heard." *Who speaks* is a central question in the cross-disciplinary, developing literature on race (Sheehi, 2021). Many BIPOC analysts and activists argue that it is their turn to speak or, more radically, that they will only speak in their own voice and have no interest in being granted a "turn to speak." And, it is not uncommon to hear White progressive analysts respond by saying, "It's my obligation to listen."

Listening, of course, is crucial. However, just waiting and listening can be problematic and paradoxical in the clinical situation, restoring the traditional, White supremacist analytic frame of "best intentions" (Hartman, 2020). Might we rethink the frame wherein the analyst must take a more activist role, lest they fall into a racialized positioning of the frame, waiting and expecting their patients of color to do the labor of introducing issues of race into the conversation? When the analyst defers to "listening," they are enacting an implicit exercise of power, which can result in silencing a patient of color in regard to issues of race and racism. (See L. Sheehi, 2021 on "psychoanalytic innocence," which "mobilizes *internally* against disequilibrium, 'innocently' excavating our own pain in order to deflect from the disruption that is unfolding.")

As Powell (2018) writes:

> Silence regarding otherness, particularly regarding race and culture, threatens every facet of our field. It is not enough to wait until others bring up these topics to engage with them. We are charged to make contact (Powell, 2018, p. 1044).

I will argue, in this chapter, that as psychoanalysts, we must step into our discomfort and wrestle with our shame and shared vulnerability, the ways in which we are all implicated; again, not equally, but meaningfully. I will emphasize the crucial imperative for White analysts, in particular, of struggling with our inclination toward silence, complicity and dissociation (Grand, 2018; Powell, 2018; Suchet, 2004). If we wait, expecting our patients of color to bring up issues of race, if we shy away, refrain from asking about racialized experience that isn't yet being named, I believe the therapy will have a superficial, as-if quality, foreclosing deeper, painful, necessarily unsettling work.

Through clinical encounters as a White analyst working with three women of color, I will investigate particular conflicts and demands that position a White therapist in a mixed-race dyad. I will examine how the internalization of racialized trauma and shame is embedded and enacted in the transference/countertransference, expanding these notions beyond the intrapsychic and relational, considering analyst and patient as unavoidably rooted in our own sociocultural, historical, and intergenerational matrix (of racial, class, gendered, and intersectional experiences), in dialogue with the other. I think here of Michelle Stephens (2021), who poetically "re-imagines the psychoanalytic encounter ... as two subjects together on an archipelagic island, where overlapping and interlapping waves of relation keep shifting the shorelines between them."

In Chapter Two, I wrote about the powerful impact of shame on the analytic process, how shame can deaden spontaneity, imagination, and creativity (Levine, 2012). In this chapter, I want to build on ways in which shame, in patient or analyst, can lead to dissociation and a focus on the self—a desire to shut down or hide; or alternatively, create an opening, an unsettled space out of which something new can emerge. When shame can be held, reflected upon, and metabolized, it can serve as a potential window into new, deeper conversations, and lead to ethical action and reparation, as Layton (2019) suggests, when inevitable racialized collisions occur. Moving closer into shame entails a willingness to step into vulnerability, letting go of one's ego, embracing the experience of the other.

Layton (2019) encourages White analysts, "not to bypass deserved shame but to move closer into it ... into an awareness of benefitting from racial inequities (which) can lead to feeling a real concern for the other, to remorse, and most importantly, to ethical action" (p. 262). Along these lines, Grand (2018) suggests, collective racial shame can feel persecutory, collapsing into violence, denial or vengeance, OR it "can be a call to conscience, an awakening to social pathologies … anticipating movement: from moralism to ethics, from solipsism to I-Thou conversation, from denial to collective responsibility" (p. 86).

I also want to build and expand on my writing, in Chapter Four, about mutual vulnerability (Levine, 2016), highlighting the shared vulnerability inherent in attending to issues of race in cross-racial analytic dyads, while holding an awareness of the asymmetries in the analytic relationship, and the complex power dynamics in racial hierarchies. I believe this entails allowing oneself to be open, challenged, and destabilized by addressing issues of race, power, and shame in the analytic relationship. In any given moment, this may deepen or disrupt the therapeutic process, dysregulating both parties, but potentially opening the possibility for honest, open dialogue.

The clinical stories I will describe underscore ways in which we need to lean into Bryan Stevenson's (2014) call to "get proximate" to suffering, reflecting on ways in which race and privilege affect our lived experience and interactions, consciously and unconsciously. I write with the understanding that, as a White analyst, I can only aim to get *psychically* proximate to race-based violence, whereas my Black, Brown and Asian patients exist in a society in which they are perpetually in danger, both physically and psychically. I try to listen for, witness, and help my patients bear trauma, including racialized trauma, paying close attention to moments of anxiety or fraught silence. I struggle with ways in which my feeling implicated in White supremacy and privilege can cause me to shut down and dissociate in moments when I wish to be present and affectively engaged.

Writing this chapter, I was struck by the complexity of attuning to race without centering Whiteness—my own White subjectivity—or objectifying or appropriating Blackness. Perhaps, in a certain sense, writing about patients is inherently incomplete and appropriative, as I believe the narrative of our therapeutic journey belongs to both of us. I'm only telling one side of the story, from my own perspective, although I aim to capture both the deep connection I feel with each of my patients and the ongoing challenges to go deeper into uncomfortable territory, and to interrogate the barriers between us.

Dionne Powell (2018) challenges us:

> How attuned are we as clinicians, as fellow citizens, to the
> collective tragedy that is racism in America, as reflected in the
> clinical situation, but also within us? To imaginatively embody,
> and vicariously hold and contain, the trauma of another is the
> daily task of psychoanalysts.
>
> (Powell, 2018, p. 1023)

Powell's article is a compelling call to action. It is a crucial challenge for
White analysts, to vicariously embody, hold and contain the racial
trauma and grief of our BIPOC patients, to recognize the limits of our
understanding and experience, and be mindful of our efforts "to restore
psychic equilibrium in unsettled White psyches" (Layton, 2019, p. 1).

In her extraordinary article, "The Condition of Black Life Is One
of Mourning," written after the 2015 Charleston massacre of nine
Black churchgoers by Dylan Roof, a White supremacist, Claudia
Rankine (2020) wrote:

> Anti-Black racism is in the culture; it's in our laws, in our
> advertisements, in our friendships, in our segregated cities, in our
> schools, in our Congress, in our scientific experiments, in our
> language, in our bodies, no matter our race, in our communities,
> and perhaps most devastatingly, in our justice system … The
> Black Lives Matter movement can be read as an attempt to keep
> mourning as an open dynamic in our culture because Black lives
> exist in a state of precariousness.

Claudia Rankine's potent assertion, about the importance of keeping
"mourning as an open dynamic in our culture because Black lives
exist in a state of precariousness," reverberates in my work with
Ruby, a Black infectious disease doctor.

"I imagine I'll cry all the way there, and all the way back," my usually
unsentimental patient, Ruby, tells me in the early weeks of Covid when
New York City had suddenly become the epicenter of the pandemic.
Ruby had just had her second child, and her department chair, a White
man, was calling her back five weeks early from maternity leave to

supervise physicians from other disciplines who had stepped in to help with the COVID-19 crisis overwhelming the hospital.

"You don't become an infectious disease doc if you don't like intense situations," Ruby says, sounding more like the Ruby I had come to know. I knew this about Ruby's career choice before the pandemic; that becoming an infectious disease doctor was a reflection of her fierce determination and fortitude that had served as an adaptive coping strategy in weathering her history of traumatic losses and the cumulative stresses of intergenerational trauma.

In our first months together, I tried to make space for Ruby to mourn, to breathe, respecting the crucial importance of her life-long defenses, enabling her to keep moving, striving, excelling. Slowly, Ruby shared grief she had never dared immersing herself in, afraid of opening the floodgates, drowning in her sorrow. When Ruby was a teenager, her beloved older sister died suddenly, leaving a hole in Ruby's heart. Then, her mother died soon after the birth of Ruby's firstborn, life and death tragically entangled. Ruby was devastated, but kept moving forward, taking care of others, a pillar of strength and resilience. This was her role in her family, the resilient one who held everyone together, a source of pride and resentment.

"I don't actually worry about getting sick myself," Ruby tells me. I am shocked, yet not shocked to hear this. I know Ruby, and this is her way. Yet there are cracks in this narrative. "But what if I get sick and spread it to my husband or kids. Part of me thinks I should quarantine from them while I'm working in the ICU. But I couldn't survive without seeing my babies." Ruby is a loving and devoted mom, and this feels like an unbearable dilemma.

Ruby: "I feel like different parts of me are at odds with each other. I feel so guilty leaving my kids, but I feel guilty not being in the hospital. This is what I'm trained to do. I'm needed there. Part of me is even excited to go back." Then, a sudden shift in self-states. "But Lauren, I'm so immersed in being a mommy right now. I can't even imagine not having Joy's newborn smell with me all the time." Ruby starts to cry. "I'm nursing her right now. This is so stressful."

Like Ruby, I am aware of powerful self-state shifts in me too: empathy, fear, concern for Ruby and her family, envy, compassion, and vulnerability. Listening to Ruby's angst about caring for patients dying from this contagious virus stirs up my own fears of getting sick, and shame that I would not want to put myself at such risk, especially in that vulnerable, postpartum period. As a mother, I feel Ruby's anguish at having to relinquish the skin-to-skin contact, the bodily intimacy of breastfeeding her newborn, to tend to her patients. I am aware of envy too: wondering what the hell I'm doing to make a difference working remotely, and more safely in this pandemic, envious of Ruby's willingness to "get proximate," *to do something* crucial that saves lives. I feel concerned about the emotional toll of her work, the trauma she is absorbing in a hospital without enough ventilators, overrun with patients, many of whom Ruby cannot save.

We, analysts and patients, are living with the deep grief and shared vulnerability of this brutal pandemic. Layers upon layers of loss, looming over us all: The unending threat of infection and death. Jobs lost, lives deferred. Graduations, weddings, and funerals conducted via Zoom. Patients' and analysts' earlier traumas triggered, spilling over into our fragilely constructed, Zoom-mediated consulting rooms. Yet, we are not at equal risk. I am working virtually, while Ruby feels compelled- even excited- to dive into the abyss, to risk her life to try to save others.

At the height of the pandemic, while Ruby was torn between the strain of the hospital and the needs of her children, my husband and older son and I drove to Colorado, where my younger son lives. It was terrifying *and thrilling* to escape the horror and dread engulfing New York City. I felt guilty, *and deeply grateful* for the privilege of leaving the city. We went speeding across the country—going 94 mph in Nebraska—where we were stopped by a White state trooper, given a huge ticket and yelled at for bringing Covid to Nebraska. This cop hated us for being New Yorkers, but didn't arrest us, or become violent. I felt grateful for my privilege, and ashamed for abusing it, negligently endangering others, and unafraid of being targeted by the police, as a White family in this very White state of Nebraska.

Our work deepens. Ruby tells me other stories, racialized stories, about life in the hospital, about the privileged White families of her patients calling frequently about their dying loved ones, suggesting experimental treatments, questioning Ruby's authority and expertise, and then reaching out to the White, male head of the hospital. I cringe listening to these stories, furious at the disrespect of these wealthy White families. I empathize with Ruby, share her rage at their audacity. Yet, privately, I wonder what I would do if one of my sons became deathly ill from COVID-19. I imagine feeling terrified, helpless, *desperate* to do anything to save my child, falling back on my privilege and access to high-quality medical care. Race and class, intermingling. I do not share these thoughts with Ruby. I wonder where they live in the space between us.

Then, after the height of the crisis in New York City, Ruby and I talk about the impact of absorbing so much trauma. Ruby tells me it felt powerful to be in Zoom meetings with her colleagues, trained to be stoic in the face of illness and death. She felt pained, witnessing their unusual expression of grief and anguish, reeling from the trauma of trying to save desperately ill patients. Yet, Ruby could not allow herself to cry, to share the depth of her trauma with her mostly White colleagues. It felt way too exposing, as one of the only Black doctors in her department. How could she dare open the door to all that grief? Grief that was both shared and separate, as a Black doctor traumatized by the collective strain of failing to save innumerable patients, and the rage, indignities and exhaustion of racial battle fatigue (Sue et al., 2019)?

I ask Ruby how it feels to share her grief with me. She tells me that sometimes it's easier than others, that she trusts me, feels my caring and support, that she can be more open with me now than at the beginning of our work together when she wasn't sure how comfortable she was going to feel opening up to a White woman. I ask about moments when it has felt harder to share her experiences around race and racism with me. She hesitates, and then responds: "Well, actually, remember when I was telling you about those families of patients dying in the ICU who were so disrespectful, going around me to complain to the head of the hospital?" I say yes, I remember. "Well, some of those families were Jewish, and that didn't feel comfortable sharing with you, knowing that you're Jewish, and not knowing how you'd react, or if you'd be offended." I ask how she was able to share that with me now. She says she wasn't sure, but that when I asked her about times that were harder to be open with me, that came immediately to mind. Then I shared with Ruby that I had actually had a feeling that they might have been Jewish, or at least some of them, and that I had felt both furious at them on her behalf, and ashamed of their entitlement and racism, doubly so if they were Jewish. I told

Ruby that not only wasn't I offended, but that I appreciated her honesty, and that she trusted me, and us, enough to share that, even if she worried about my reaction. I am aware of how much I miss seeing Ruby in person, the presence of our two bodies in the room together, and I wonder with her how working virtually affects our sense of closeness, intimacy, anxiety and our struggle to "construct necessary scaffolding to bridge the cross-racial divide" (Vaughans, 2022) between us.

In the next session, we talked about Ruby's sense of exhaustion, the trauma of caring for COVID patients, and being yanked away from her newborn, feeling like she is failing in both realms, impossibly stretched and split between her babies and the demands of the ICU. This was in the midst of the protests following George Floyd's murder. Ruby continued:

> I'm exhausted. And I feel kind of numb about this overdue White reckoning with racism. Why do Black Lives Matter now? What's taken so long? Every White person I've ever known is texting me to say she's thinking of me, telling me what she told her White kids about the George Floyd murder and police brutality against Black boys and men, and by the way, "What should she be reading to educate herself?

"I don't even feel like responding," Ruby adds. "Why are you looking to me to do the work for you? *White Fragility* and *How to be an Anti-Racist* are on the bestseller lists. Educate *yourself.*"

I am struck by this unusually open expression of anger on Ruby's part, and ask her what it's like to talk with me, her White therapist, about this. "Oh, it's fine," she responds, way too quickly. "I could talk about race all day. I grew up talking about race." I wonder what's not being said, what Ruby finds hard to say, what I find hard to ask, to hear. Ruby grew up talking about race with Black folks, not White folks. I wonder how free Ruby feels to share her rage— unapologetically—with me, worried about my capacity to take it in without anxiety or defensiveness. But I don't say more in this moment. I hold back, unsure how to inquire directly, to wonder with Ruby about how it might not be easy or fine to talk with me about her rage over daily, cumulative experiences with racism. It's only later, after the session, that I hear the transferential messages loud and clear, realizing I did not think to ask in the moment, "Do you ever feel anything like this with me, *like I look to you to do the work for me?*"

I realize it will take time to keep developing a deeper trust, living through enactments and reparations, to build the stamina to survive ruptures and honest reckonings around mis-attunements regarding race. I listen carefully, pay attention to both verbal and non-verbal cues, for moments when I sense Ruby (or myself) holding back, not delving deeper into the pain, rage, and shame of *micro-aggressions* and overt racism that she has absorbed over a lifetime.

Ruby tells me she can talk about race all day, that she grew up talking about race. I however, did not. Or, I should say, as a White, Jewish, upper middle-class daughter of progressive parents, I grew up very aware of race and racism. My parents were actively involved in social justice work, and my Jewish identity was strongly linked to social action. But I had no real racialized consciousness of my Whiteness and internalized racism, no words to describe the privilege of my Whiteness. I remember feeling guilty about my Whiteness and economic privilege, or more accurately, what Mitchell described as "guiltiness," which he differentiates from true guilt.

Mitchell (2000) suggests that genuine guilt entails an acceptance of accountability for suffering we have caused others. "Without genuine guilt, we cannot risk loving, because the terror of our destructiveness is too great … Guilt needs to be distinguished from … 'guiltiness'— perpetual payments in an internal protection racket that can never end" (p. 731). Guiltiness is characterized more by self-pity. "By making static, private arrangements with ourselves around self-pity and guilt, we close ourselves off from engaging a world of other people in which the risks, as well as the potential rewards, are enormous" (p. 732).

It has taken me years to directly acknowledge the ways in which I have benefited from White privilege, to grapple with the moral imperative of being implicated in oppressive systems of White supremacy. Over time, as I have come into leadership positions, I have felt the responsibility, urgency, and empowerment to prioritize anti-racism efforts, to address inequities and injustices in our analytic spaces.

Reading DiAngelo's book, *White Fragility* cracked something open in me, gave me language to describe some of what I had felt for years, but had not had the words for, to look at my internalized racism and White privilege with less anxiety and defensiveness. But, recognizing myself in her descriptions was a destabilizing journey, as I shifted from recognition to disavowal, traversing an internal process of trying, failing, and trying again to reckon with my White fragility. I cringed at DiAngelo's critique of White progressive imagination and intentions. Working to own my own biases, I felt myself slowly taking in her words, acknowledging my guiltiness and efforts to prove myself and my virtuosity. It felt by turns daunting and liberating to recognize myself in DiAngelo's words, to metabolize my shame, as a White progressive who saw myself as someone from a family with "good values." Reading *White Fragility* helped me move out of immobilizing guiltiness, toward what Grand calls, "creative shame" that "increases our awareness of the other, restores our humanity, begins a movement toward restorative justice." This is ongoing work for us White folks to confront our own racism, to acknowledge and bear witness to the destructive impact of our internalized bias and privilege, and repair the inevitable collisions that will occur when we are open to having these conversations.

Ruby and I have talked about the precariousness of the bodies of Black boys and men (Vaughans, 2016), and she has expressed terror about the dangers that her son will face as a teenager and young adult. She worries about her active, high-spirited young son, going to preschool for the first time, afraid of how White teachers will treat him, whether they will single him out as "bad" or "wild." On the other hand, she worries that maybe she disciplines him too harshly, to teach him to be calmer and more self-contained, out of fear of White teachers overreacting and punishing him more severely than his White peers.

Here, I am mindful of Claudia Rankine again:

> Though the White liberal imagination likes to feel temporarily bad about black suffering, there really is no mode of empathy that can replicate the daily strain of knowing that as a black person you can be killed for simply being black: No hands in your pockets, no playing music, no sudden movements, no driving your car, no walking at night, no walking in the day, ... no standing your ground, no standing here, no standing there.

Recently, Ruby told me a story about walking in the park with her young son, who is short for his age. A White man walking by said, "Oh, he's so cute. He's going to be a basketball player when he grows up." Ruby noted plaintively to me, "They never say, 'He's going to be a chemist.'" A moment later, she added, "But, it's fine." "But it's *not* fine," I countered. Ruby immediately pivoted: "Right, it's *not* fine. It's enraging actually. It's *infuriating*. Things like that happen all the time." I asked Ruby what made her say initially that it was "fine?" She responded, "Everyday I have encounters where I have to decide, should I deal with this or let it go? You know, either way, it's *exhausting*. You can't possibly respond to every micro-aggression. I'd be furious all the time." I try to feel my way into this impossible dilemma Ruby describes, imagining the toll it would take to feel the rage each time I experienced a racial affront, or a "stereotypical, defensive, hyper-masculine" racist projection of a Black male directed to one of my sons (Vaughans and Spielberg, 2014). To respond directly, or push it down. Because it's too hard and draining to react every time. It's a double bind, with a pernicious, cumulative impact.

While this conversation opened space for us to reflect on Ruby's rage, I didn't ask how *Ruby felt* in response to this man's racism. I responded with my own outrage. But I didn't go deeper, or ask Ruby to go deeper. In joining Ruby in her *outrage*, purportedly on *her* behalf, *perhaps I was avoiding my own White shame*, disavowing any identification with this White man and his racist stereotypes. *Not me. Not me.* Projection allowing the enemy to be located *outside*. What made Ruby say it was "fine" at first? Who was the "fine" for, for me, for her? Where does disavowed rage live in Ruby, and in our work together? How safe does Ruby feel to express rage with me or toward me, to trust that we can survive and manage intense conflict and rage? How safe does it feel *to me to ask?* I wonder how to make more space for transferential rage—rage directed at me—and to risk being the oppressor, the bad object with regard to enactments around race. I wonder about overlaps and differences in our lives, our shared grief and shared rage, and about the limits of my White subjectivity, my capacity, in Powell's words, to "imaginatively embody, and vicariously hold and contain" Ruby's racialized trauma. I care deeply about Ruby, and I want to stretch the limits of my understanding and witnessing. I aspire to a deeper level of *sturdiness* in regard to discussing issues of race and racism.

I am inspired by what Garth Stevens (2020) writes about both unbridgeable gaps and possibilities for connection in working clinically with racialized trauma:

> There are indeed limits to the processes of knowing, recognition, comprehensibility, and resolution, but these limits can themselves offer opportunities for continued accompaniment and generativity, with ongoing possibilities for psychic reorganization, recalibration and change for both therapists and patients (p. 721).

George Floyd's murder was a tipping point for some White Americans, belatedly waking up to the pervasive violence and horror of systemic racism. But, as Soraya Nadia McDonald, in her trenchant piece, "The dangerous magical thinking of 'This is not who we are,'" noted,

> The truth is all around us. It was all around us before George Floyd, before Breonna Taylor, before Ahmaud Arbery, before Atatiana Jefferson, before Trayvon Martin, before Emmett Till, before Recy Taylor, before Mary Turner, before J. Marion Sims, the "father of gynecology" who repeatedly butchered enslaved women named Lucy, Anarcha and Betsey without anesthesia.
>
> (McDonald, 2021)

We were blind to these devastating truths, preferring the defensive notion, as White progressives, that "This is not who we are" (Caflisch, 2020), exempting ourselves from culpability and reckoning.

For Black Americans, the pernicious effect of racism has been an ongoing source of "weathering," a term coined by Dr. Arline Geronimus, who has been studying the impact of racism on Black bodies for over thirty years. Weathering is meant to evoke a sense of *erosion* from the chronic stress of living in a racist society, the physiological impact down to the cellular level—a premature aging of the cells, causing higher levels of inflammation and disease—caused by the everyday lived experience of racism. In an episode of the podcast, *The United States of Anxiety*, "Why Covid 19 is Killing Black People" (April, 24, 2020), Kai Wright interviews Dr. Geronimus about the impact of weathering on Black peoples' bodies and psyches; connected to the vast disparities in African-American vulnerability to Covid, in addition to disparate access to health care, greater numbers of BIPOC individuals working as front-line workers, and racism embedded in our medical system. They discuss the complexity of resilience for African-American people, both the individual and collective strength and stamina that has allowed them to survive the long arc of slavery, Jim Crow, lynchings, redlining, and its current manifestations in anti-Black violence, mass incarceration, and the physiological and psychological toll it takes to endure racism in all its malignant forms.

I have been seeing Angela, a Caribbean-American woman, for several years, initially for anxiety and self-esteem issues. Angela is a warm, outgoing person, involved in her church, highly educated, and successful in her career. We talk often about books we're reading, politics, race, and the horrors of the Trump presidency. After the 2020 election, we discussed our shared relief and a renewed sense of lightness; a desire to be hopeful, but not naïve about the weight of history and the massive need for change in our country.

Then, when Trump incited millions to question the validity of the election and tried to disenfranchise BIPOC voters, and yet another unarmed Black man was murdered, Angela told me: "My parents taught me, as a Black woman, I had to work harder, be better. But Lauren, I'm *tired!* I feel like moving my Black children back to the Islands, where it feels safer and more homey," where Angela's parents were raised, surrounded by other Black folks. Angela comes from a long legacy of strong Black women and mothers, from whom, she tells me, she learned how to be a mother to her children, a fierce defender and protector. She yearns to create a refuge for her family, a sense of safety and belonging, a respite from the ongoing stress of violent racism. I am acutely aware of my White privilege in that moment when Angela tells me about her desperate desire to keep her children safe by taking them back to the islands, when I have driven out to Colorado with my family.

Angela tells me she grew up in a neighborhood of mostly Black and Brown folks and is grateful for the refuge and sense of belonging that her neighborhood, school, and church provided, which she fervently wants to provide her own children. She wants to give them the best education possible, and wonders, with her husband, whether to spend the money to send them to private school, whether it would be worth the cost—and the psychic cost to her children—of being one of the few Black children in their class.

Then, Angela tells me something she had not told me before, which takes me by surprise; that she has always felt suspicious of White people and their intentions. This feels significant, that she can now trust me, and the resilience of our relationship enough to reveal this. She shares that she had felt skeptical about seeing a White therapist when we began working together, unsure of whether she could talk freely about her experiences as a Black woman, whether I would "get it," and especially whether or not I would feel comfortable talking about race. She remembers the turning point early on, when I asked her whether an experience at work felt racist, which led to a more open conversation about race in which I asked how she felt working with a White therapist. I remember her responding, "Oh it's fine, my friend (who is Black), who referred me to you told me you were White, but you were cool."

Clearly, it had not felt cool *before* that initial conversation, which Angela and I now laughed about, as it had taken time to speak more candidly. Angela was understandably cautious about my openness and comfort talking about race, and had not mentioned race at all previously. In this recent conversation, she remembered feeling relieved that I brought up race directly, and said that that had felt important to her, let her know I was up for talking about race. But I had to work hard to gain her trust, before we could have deeper, more direct racial conversations.

I wonder, however, where the suspicion of White folks lives in the therapy, why Angela brought it up at this moment. What was she communicating? Was she concerned about my reaction to her impulse to take her children away from this racist country, to the safer, homey Islands surrounded by other Black folks? How much does she feel the need to protect me, and our relationship? How much does our mutual need to protect the trust we've built inhibit our capacity to raise questions that go further, deeper? And what are the costs of dissociating the doubts, suspicions, aggression, and hurt of not feeling deeply seen and understood?

After the violent White supremacist insurrection on January 6, Angela felt wracked with fear and grief about how unsafe this country feels for her family. I felt horrified and enraged by the riot at the Capitol, and resonated with Angela's devastation. But in this session, I felt unusually muted, frozen, immobilized. I struggled to think, to put my strong feelings into words. I did not know whether my internal struggle was apparent to Angela. But I felt a deep sense of shame afterwards that I had felt silenced, dissociated, unable to stay connected to Angela in her anguish. Reflecting on the session later, I realized I had hesitated, questioned whether I had a right to fully share her grief, given my Whiteness and privilege. I felt ashamed of our country's history, about the insidious impact of Trump's lies and inciting of White supremacist violence and attempted coup. I resonated with Knoblauch (2020), a White analyst's description of his experience with his Black patient, Waverly,

> trying to balance on the cliff-like edge of an uncanny (socially constructed) gap ... that cannot be traversed ... a place in clinical encounter where training fails as a refuge for mentalization and emotional balance, a point of urgency opening up into opportunity. (p. 304)

In our next session, I asked Angela how she had felt in our last meeting and shared some of my experience with her. I wondered aloud with her about what had prevented me from engaging more openly about my horror about the insurrection, a hesitation from empathizing more fully with her. I apologized for holding back, sharing the ways in which I felt implicated, complicit, as a White American. Angela was visibly moved, and said she appreciated my openness and vulnerability, my willingness to reflect on my Whiteness and shame. Then she became more curious about my background. Had I grown up in New York City (like her)? What were my family's religion and politics, and were any of my relatives Trump supporters? I responded that it felt important to her to know more about me, my family, where my people came from. I was open with her, answered questions that she had not felt comfortable asking earlier, or perhaps had not wondered about at all. I wondered with her what it was like to ask and know these parts of my family and identity. Angela told me that I was among a small handful of White folks she felt close to, felt she could trust, that she could let her guard down with me. Although she did not ask directly, I also sensed her wondering about how our histories and identities overlapped and diverged, what we had in common, how our lives differed. Angela knows that I have two grown sons and will sometimes ask me about my experiences parenting boys, now young men, if I still worry about them. She says she senses that I am a protective "mama bear" like her. We have talked about the differences raising Black boys with the attendant parental terrors that they could be arrested, shot or killed just for being Black. I experienced her queries as efforts to locate me socio-culturally, to probe and reach me, expanding on Winnicott and Ghent's (1990) notions of probing, or object finding as an effort to reach and recognize, to "dis-cover" another.

But I still wonder what happened in that session, in the back and forth of transference/countertransference with Angela that made me feel particularly silenced, distanced, put me in touch with my White shame about the horrors of this country, our history, and the particularly horrific experience of living through the Trump presidency. I wonder what it was in Angela's particularly tormented state of mind and the intense vulnerability she expressed as a Black woman, and mother, in the U.S. that felt hard for me to bear and hold and speak to in this session, such that I needed time to reflect, to find my bearings, find my voice, to re-connect with Angela.

I have found in my work with BIPOC patients that it's crucial for me to open conversations about race if they do not do so spontaneously, to make it clear that I am interested and up for reflecting on issues of race and power, that I want to hear about their history with White people and in White spaces, and the racial trauma embedded in those experiences. Suchet (2004) suggests, "Most patients are willing to collude in the denial of racial dynamics between patient and analyst" (p. 435). I have found that once I open the conversation, once I make it clear that I'm comfortable hearing and engaging issues of race—or if not always comfortable, then willing to step into the discomfort—to be challenged about my own biases and blind-spots, and *to listen*—then people speak much more openly about a lifetime of experiences of racism and micro-aggressions, what it's like for them to live as a Black or Brown person in America. But this openness waxes and wanes, easier with some patients than others, as we each struggle to share our most vulnerable selves, our biases and anxieties across racial divides.

Heather, who is Navajo on her mother's side, grew up aware of her Native history, yet knew little about it, often passing as White. She has not been confronted by racism directed at her on a daily basis. Yet, racial trauma takes different, complex, embodied forms. Heather came to therapy struggling with depression and anxiety – and a sense, as far back as she can remember, that something was wrong with her, that her feelings and reactions were too intense, that she cries too easily and often, and doesn't know why. Her mother grew up on a reservation and is loath to talk about her traumatic personal history, or the history of her people. Heather is proud of her Navajo identity, but she has become even more anxious to hear stories about her Native history since George Floyd's murder.

Heather told me about a podcast she had just discovered about Native identity and history called, *All Our Relations*, which had a potent impact on her. She described how the eighty-minute conversation between two Indigenous hosts went by in a flash, as she has been hungry for more knowledge and understanding about her Navajo identity. She tells me it felt enormously comforting, like having conversations she has never had, but always wished she could have with her mother. She bought a book on Native history that sat unopened on her night table. As she and I have been talking more about her Navajo history, she began reading, and then could not stop. She told me how devastating it has been reading stories of American colonists massacring Native people. "This isn't the history we're taught. We don't read or talk about the extent of the violence, the wiping out of families and communities. Why aren't we taught the whole truth of what happened to my people??" Heather cried.

Learning more about her peoples' devastating history, hearing the voices and stories of two fellow Indigenous women opened access to a depth of emotion that shook Heather to her core. This opened a door to the impact of intergenerational trauma, a door sealed shut over generations, reminiscent of Abraham and Torok's (1984) notion of endocryptic identification, the creation of a haunted, closed-off space, a *crypt,* around a gaping wound—a ghostly identification with a traumatically lost object (p. 223). For the first time, Heather was able to open the door to the crypt, step warily in, and explore forbidden territory from her ancestral past, together. We reflected on how she has been carrying the weight of unprocessed trauma, throughout her life, in her body. Over many sessions, Heather cried and cried, years of tears, for her mother's and grandmother's unmourned trauma. Heather tells me,

> Most of my relatives are dead. I don't even know if I have aunts, uncles and cousins who are still alive, whose stories are lost to me. My mom is the only one who knows these stories. She's the storykeeper. But they're my stories too.

I tell Heather how excruciating this feels, to sense the deep wounds of her mother, and her ancestors' genocide, without knowing their actual stories. Then, haunted by ghostly transgenerational trauma, these conversations stirred questions about parts of my own family history that had been erased, dissociated. I had always thought we didn't have family killed in the Holocaust. I never questioned this until these discussions with Heather. We were discussing how Indigenous children were forced by the U.S. government to attend residential schools to rid them of their Native identity and customs and the thousands of children murdered and discovered in mass graves. Suddenly, this jolted me into associations to the millions of Jews forced into concentration camps, slaughtered by the Nazis. How was it possible that I had no relatives killed in the Holocaust, when my Jewish ancestors were mostly from Poland, where 3.3 million Jews lived before the war, more than any other country in Europe, and only 380,000 remained alive in 1945? So I face-timed my great Aunt Harriet, the only living relative of my grandparent's generation, the *storykeeper* of our family. She confirmed that while we had no *known* relatives murdered in the Holocaust, there was family left behind, with whom they had lost touch when my grandparents immigrated, a parallel generation most likely exterminated.

Layli Long Soldier (2021), a Native poet and Lakota artist, writes,

> We remember who we are from our families, from this land, from stories within the community, and from our senses. Yet, from our senses, we remember what's stored within us already. Maybe/ sometimes, I/we cannot put words to it, but we feel something ... I might call it instinct. It's an old sensation that cannot be named, for which there is no textual record or language to help us understand. Yet it is there just below the skin. (pp. 57–58)

In the next session, Heather tells me that she has had a startlingly open conversation with her mom about growing up on the reservation. Heather says,

> I never would have dared broaching that conversation with my mom if we hadn't been talking about all this. But it was important, essential even. Things that have never made sense to me are falling into place. Like why I was depressed as a teenager. No one knew why. Even I didn't know. Everyone assumed it was biochemical. But no one thought to ask me about all this, my Native family trauma.

These conversations helped Heather feel less crazy, alone and isolated. It has felt important to help Heather be gentler on herself, understanding of where her intense feelings come from, that she has been carrying the wounds of history (Apprey, Salberg, Gump). Reminiscent of Henri Rey's notion that patients come into therapy to heal their parents, Heather is anxious to heal her mother's wounds. Having always felt that her mother "had suffered enough," Heather now has the courage to broach her mother's traumatic past with a sense of her right to know her cultural and intergenerational history, which is her history, her story too.

Recently, Heather described how not feeling heard or listened to is triggering, enraging to her. "Like what I say doesn't matter, like I don't matter. Like I'm invisible." She began to cry. "I don't know why this is so upsetting, bigger than the situation itself, like I get more upset than I should." Long pause. "That suddenly makes me think of Native invisibility ... I imagine my mom must have felt unheard, like there was no one there to listen, no one to hear her pain and sadness." In our work together, we are struggling to disrupt the intergenerational trauma of not mattering, *the theft* of not mattering, to feel like she matters, her *trauma* matters, her *peoples' trauma* matters. Soon afterward, Heather asked to meet more often, to go deeper into our work together.

This political moment raises crucial questions about our ethical responsibility as analysts to take the lead in bringing conversations about race into the consulting room, and, equally important, although it's not the focus of this chapter, to challenge our White patients to reflect on their privilege and Whiteness, to turn "White guilt" into meaningful action (e.g., Caflisch, 2020; Cyrus, 2020; Davids, 2020; DiAngelo, 2018; Melamed, 2021, Suchet, 2004; Straker, 2004; Swartz, 2020). Suchet (2004) suggests,

> Race haunts our consciousness. Like a melancholic structure, disavowed and unacknowledged … We need to own our racial identity and embrace a space where the horrors of trauma can be reenacted … We cannot afford to dissociate the shame and guilt we carry as a consequence of being the oppressors, historically and currently. (pp. 435–6)

Isabel Wilkerson, in her brilliant book, *Caste: The Origins of Our Discontents* writes that unaddressed prejudice and racism can cause worsened health and premature illness, and that being racist erodes White peoples' bodies too:

> The friction of caste is killing people. Societal inequity is killing people. The act of moving about and navigating spaces with those whom society has trained us to believe are inherently different from us is killing people, and not just the targets. Studies are showing that prejudice itself can be deadly. (p. 304)

White supremacy affects—*and infects*—all of us, in our bodies, in our histories, in the stories we tell, and pass down to our children and grandchildren.

Harris (2020) writes of the potential of the pandemic as a moment of "unbinding"; dangerous but holding the potential for growth and transformation. As the novelist, Arundhati Roy (2020) stresses:

> Nothing would be worse than a return to normality. Historically, pandemics have forced humans to break with the past and imagine their worlds anew. This one is no different. It is a portal, a gateway between one world and the next. We can choose to walk through it, dragging the carcasses of our prejudice and hatred, our avarice, dead ideas, dead rivers and smoky skies behind us. Or we can walk through it … ready to imagine another world.

With COVID-19 still raging, there is a collective longing for a return to "normalcy," an end to social distancing and zoom-mediated communication, a longing to hug friends and family, to begin to repair the medical, psychological, sociocultural, and socioeconomic devastation that has befallen us. But this moment calls for something more, something different. Not a return to the past, but a wake-up call for the importance of change, a belief in our fundamental interdependence and our need for each other.

As Gwendolyn Brooks urgently and poetically reminds us: "We are each other's harvest, we are each other's business; we are each other's magnitude and bond."

I am deeply grateful to Ruby, Angela, and Heather, and the patients in all the chapters, for their generosity in giving me permission to share their, and our, stories. And to all the people I work with who are visibly and invisibly similar and different from me, for all that they have taught me, and all that we have learned together on our unique and moving journeys.

References

Abraham, N. and Torok, M. (1984). "The lost object—Me:" Notes on identification within the crypt. *Psychoanalytic Inquiry*, 4: 221–242.

Caflisch, J. (2020). "When reparation Is felt to be impossible": Persecutory guilt and breakdowns in thinking and dialogue about race. *Psychoanalytic Dialogues*, 30:578–594.

Cyrus, K. (2020). When reparation *is* impossible: A discussion of "When reparation Is felt to be impossible": Persecutory guilt and breakdowns in thinking and dialogue about race. *Psychoanalytic Dialogues*, 30: 595–603.

Davids, F. (2020). Discussion of "When reparation Is felt to be impossible": Persecutory guilt and breakdowns in thinking and dialogue about race. *Psychoanalytic Dialogues*, 30: 604–612.

DiAngelo, R, (2018). *White fragility: Why it's so hard for White people to talk about racism*. Boston, MA: Beacon Press.

Edugyan, E. (2021). *Out of the sun: On race and storytelling*. Canada: House of Anansi Press.

Gay, V. (2016). *On the pleasures of owning persons: The hidden face of American slavery*. New York: International Psychoanalytic Books.

Grand, S. (2018). The other within: White shame and Native American genocide. *Contemporary Psychoanalysis*, 54: 84–102.

Harris, A. (2019). The perverse pact: Racism and White privilege. *American Imago*, 76: 309–333.

Hartman, S. (2020). Blinded by the White: A discussion of Fanon's vision of embodied racism for psychoanalytic theory and practice. *Psychoanalytic Dialogues*, 3: 317–324.

Kabasakalian-McKay, R. and Mark, D. (Eds.) (2022). *Inhabiting Implication*.

Knoblauch, S. (2020). Fanon's vision of embodied racism for psycho-analytic theory and practice. *Psychoanalytic Dialogues*, 30: 299–316.

Layton, L. (2019). Transgenerational hauntings: Toward a social psychoanalysis and an ethic of dis-illusionment. *Psychoanalytic Dialogues*, 29: 105–121.

Levine, L. (2016). A mutual survival of destructiveness and its creative potential for agency and desire. *Psychoanalytic Dialogues*, 26: 36–49.

Levine, L. (2012). Into thin air: Co-constructing shame, recognition, and creativity in an analytic process. *Psychoanalytic Dialogues*, 22: 456–471.

McDonald, S. (2021). The dangerous magical thinking of 'This is not who we are.' Web. *The Undefeated*, January 14, 2021.

Melamed, C. (2021). A White person problem: Conducting White/White treatment with a social justice lens. *Psychoanalytic Social Work*, 1–24.

Mitchell, S. (2000). You've got to suffer if you want to sing the blues: Psychoanalytic reflections on guilt and self-pity. *Psychoanalytic Dialogues*, 10, 713–733.

Nichols, B. and Connolly, M. (2020). Transforming ghosts into ancestors: Unsilencing the psychological case for reparations to descendants of American slavery.

Powell, D. (2018). Race, African Americans and psychoanalysis: Collective silence in the therapeutic conversation. *Journal of the American Psychoanalytic Association*, 66:1021–1049.

Rankine, C. (2020). The Condition of Black Life is One of Mourning. *The Sunday Read, in The Daily*, June 7, 2020.

Rothberg, M. (2019). *The implicated subject: Beyond victims and perpetrators*. Stanford CA: Stanford University Press.

Roy, A. (2020). The pandemic is a portal. *Financial Times*, April 3, 2020. https://www.ft.com/content/10d8f5e8-74eb-11ea-95fe-fcd274e920ca

Sheehi, L. (2021). Psychoanalytic innocence: The ideological underpinnings of theory and praxis. Psychology and the Other Conference, September 19, 2021.

Soldier, L.L. (2021). I cannot stop: A reminder of the murder of George Floyd. In T.K. Smith and J. Freeman (Eds) *There's a revolution outside, my love: Letters from a crisis*. Vintage Books.

Sadek, N. (in press). Racial justice in psychoanalytic communities: Translating antiracist dialogues into racial equity. *Psychoanalytic Dialogues*.

Stephens, M. (2021). On "The burning beach:" Immersion, errantry, and the Caribbean relation. *Psychoanalytic Dialogues*, 31: 593–601.

Stevens, G. (2020). Racial alienation, the (im)possibilities of resolution, and the absent/present other. *Psychoanalytic Dialogues*, 30: 716–722.

Stephens, M. (2022). Relational racialization and segregated whiteness. *Psychoanalytic Dialogues*, 32:114–120.

Stevenson, B. (2014). *Just mercy: A story of justice and redemption.* New York: Spiegel and Grau.

Straker, G. (2004). Race for cover: Castrated Whiteness, perverse consequences. *Psychoanalytic Dialogues*, 14: 405–422.

Suchet, M. (2004). A relational encounter with race. *Psychoanalytic Dialogues*, 14: 423–438.

Sue, D.W., Alsaidi, S., Awad, M.N., Glaeser, E., Calle, C.Z., and Mendez, N. (2019). Disarming racial micro-aggressions: Microintervention strategies for targets, White allies, and bystanders. *American Psychologist*, 74(1): 128–142.

Swartz, S. (2020). Giving in, giving up, and being blown to smithereens: A discussion of "When reparation Is felt to be impossible": Persecutory guilt and breakdowns in thinking and dialogue about race. *Psychoanalytic Dialogues*, 30: 613–620.

Vaughans, K. (2016). Conversations on Psychoanalysis and Race. *The American Psychoanalyst (TAP)*, 50, No.3.

Vaughans, K. and Spielberg. W. (2014). The psychology of Black boys and adolescents.

Vaughans, K. C. (2022). Commentary on Lauren Levine's "Interrogating Race, Shame and Mutual Vulnerability". *Psychoanalytic Dialogues*, 32:126–129.

Wilkerson, I. (2020). *Caste: The origins of our discontents.* New York: Random House.

Index

For Product Safety Concerns and Information please contact our EU
representative GPSR@taylorandfrancis.com
Taylor & Francis Verlag GmbH, Kaufingerstraße 24, 80331 München, Germany

9 781032 434742